# Chair Yoga for Seniors over 60

## 28 DAYS TO DOUBLE FITNESS WITH GENTLE EXERCISE

CHARLIE ATLAS

ZENWISDOM PRESS

# Contents

# Introduction

If you're reading this, chances are you've made a commitment to become healthier and you're ready to take the first step towards improving your well-being. This is an excellent decision that can make a significant difference in your life. As we grow older, it's crucial to maintain an active lifestyle and prioritize our health. Starting a new exercise routine can be daunting, particularly for people aged 60 and above. However, I want to assure you that there's no better time to get motivated and start your fitness journey. Chair yoga is an excellent starting point.

With just a few minutes of practice each day, chair yoga can significantly impact your health and general well-being. This gentle form of exercise offers seniors numerous benefits, including increased flexibility, strength, balance, and mental clarity. And the best part is that you can do it all from the comfort of your home with nothing more than a sturdy chair and a positive attitude. It's easy to underestimate the power of just a few minutes of exercise each day. Still, the truth is that even small amounts of physical activity can have a significant impact on your health. By incorporating chair yoga into your daily routine, you'll feel better physically and experience increased energy levels, reduced stress, and a greater sense of overall happiness.

As we age, we might experience a gradual decline in our physical abilities. Activities that we once found easy may now require more effort or time. Workouts might take longer; walks may become less brisk, or even simple tasks like carrying groceries might feel heavier. Initially, we might not notice these changes, but over time, they can lead to persistent discomforts and limitations.

For many of us, the fear of losing independence is a significant concern as we age. Mobility issues may force us to stay home to avoid slowing others down or risking falls. This isolation can lead to feelings of depression and pose threats to our mental well-being. We all strive to maintain our connections with loved ones while preserving our independence, but achieving it can be challenging.

This is where low-impact chair yoga comes in as a gentle and accessible form of exercise that can help to alleviate these concerns. When practiced regularly, the simple exercises in this 28-day routine can help to improve mobility, maintain balance, enhance flexibility, and double your fitness. This, in turn, enables us to sustain our independent lifestyle for years to come.

Before dismissing chair yoga as unsuitable, let's dispel some misconceptions. Yoga isn't solely about contorting into challenging poses; it's about fostering a connection with oneself, one's body, and the surrounding environment. Whether you're looking to relieve chronic pain, boost your mood, or stay active and independent as you age, chair yoga offers a simple and effective solution. Let's take the first step toward a healthier, happier, and more vibrant you.

Chair yoga is designed to cater to individuals with various needs and abilities. It emphasizes starting small, celebrating progress, and gradually building strength and confidence. While some may initially feel apprehensive about the spiritual aspects associated with yoga, what truly matters is its tangible benefits. The focus should be on the effectiveness of the exercises rather than their cultural origins.

Imagine a tailored routine that respects your unique needs and progresses at a pace that suits you, ensuring you feel empowered rather than overwhelmed.

We believe that within 28 days, you can double your fitness. This doesn't mean that you will be able to lift twice the amount of weight or move twice as fast, but 28 days is enough time to transform your body and rejuvenate your outlook on life. A regimen that's straightforward yet remarkably effective, leaving you wondering why you didn't embark on this journey sooner. That's the essence of chair yoga, and this book isn't just a mere guide—it's a roadmap meticulously crafted to fast-track your journey toward a healthier, more independent life.

Before we dive into the exercises, we'll provide you with a comprehensive understanding of chair yoga—its origins, purpose, and why it's an ideal fit for you, addressing your specific needs. We'll guide you through setting up your practice space, ensuring it's safe, comfortable, and conducive to productive sessions. Efficient breathing techniques will be emphasized, showcasing how mindful breathing can lead to relaxation and enhanced well-being.

Furthermore, we'll lead you through a step-by-step routine to restore your confident posture, introducing gentle exercises that promote increased flexibility and overall mobility while gradually building muscle strength to enhance stability and reduce the risk of falls. As a result, you'll feel more capable and secure in your daily activities.

We will address sleep, a crucial overlooked aspect, and highlight its significance in stress reduction and overall health. We'll provide exercises to promote restful, rejuvenating sleep every night.

We will discuss any concerns you may have related to focus and memory, which can be a norm of aging that you don't necessarily have to follow. We'll introduce chair yoga movements that help maintain sharpness and agility, mitigating common age-related challenges. Additionally, we'll discuss the vital role of nutrition in bolstering strength, energy, mental acuity, and pain management, offering practical tips to complement your chair yoga practice with nourishing dietary choices.

Finally, we'll consolidate everything into a concise 28-day plan, which, when followed correctly, can double your fitness, increase mobility, maintain balance, and improve flexibility.

Embark on this transformative journey with us—acquiring knowledge and embracing transformation. Each step serves as a building block, and every chapter is a stepping stone toward the vibrant, active life we aspire to. If you're ready to redefine aging, rediscover your zest for life, and embark on a rejuvenated journey, then welcome to your transformation.

Before you begin, if the images in this book are too small, please scan this QR code with your phone camera to download larger pictures and the full movement chart.

# How to use this book

The aim of this book is to get you fitter, quicker with no injuries, and help you arrive at your goal with a better mindset. Used correctly it will improve your life.

First things first.

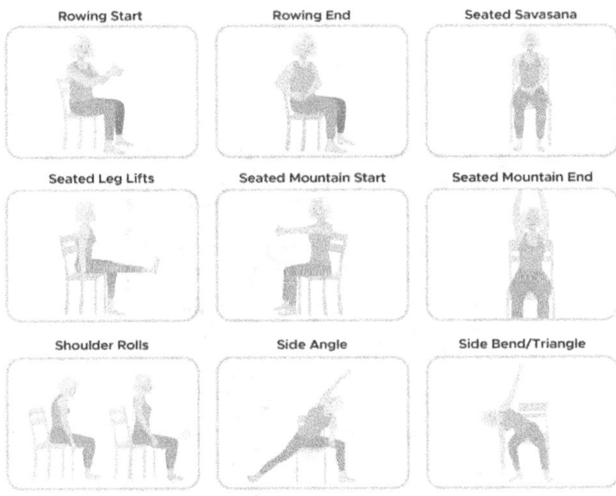

This book is filled with exercise illustrations that you can follow easily, but if they are too small or not clear enough, please download our free reference chart here https://f2edg3.systeme.io/zenwisdompress. Or scan the QR code below. You don't need to provide any information to get the chart, so you can safely download it or print it out to help master the movements.

We suggest:

Please read the book and follow along; at first, you may have to read a section, put your book down, and do the exercise, but after a couple of times, you will know how each exercise is done, and you won't need the book. Try to Do the fitness test before the 28-day routine; this will give you a starting point to show you how much you've improved. The exercises are gentle enough to do immediately, take your time, and you will improve daily.

Exercises in the book won't be practical if not performed correctly, so try to get your form right by diligently following the routines and advice outlined here. As with any exercise routine, you must consult your doctor before beginning this chair yoga regimen if you have pre-existing conditions. Please send us your questions or suggestions through our website www.ZenWisdomPress.net, and don't forget to leave us a quick Amazon review when you're done reading so that others can discover Chair Yoga for themselves. Scan The Code below for your free Chart.

# What is Chair Yoga?

"Age is an issue of mind over matter. If you don't mind, it doesn't matter." – Mark Twain

Chair Yoga is a great way to get fit. It's very flexible for people who struggle with movement, helping them regain flexibility and retrieve more movement. Older adults seem to choose chair yoga because it's easy to do and works.

Everyone's body starts to get worn out as they age; very few people can say that they don't have at least some aches and pains. Chair yoga provides a solution to these challenges. Instead of complex poses on gym mats, a simple dining room chair suffices, offering necessary support without the strain of challenging floor positions. When performed correctly, chair yoga can deliver many of the same benefits as traditional yoga exercises.

At its core, chair yoga can bring people together. It's yoga that anyone can partake in, whether from the comfort of home or even the office.

You don't need to be exceptionally flexible or have prior yoga experience. All required is a chair and the willingness to move and stretch.

While it may initially seem like a modern adaptation or a diluted version of traditional yoga, chair yoga is a potent and accessible modification designed to extend yoga's profound benefits to those finding traditional poses challenging or impractical.

So, what exactly is chair yoga, and what will we expect you to do? It incorporates true elements of traditional yoga, breathing exercises, poses, and meditation, which is tailored to be performed while seated or with the support of a chair. This adaptation ensures that even individuals finding prolonged standing or floor-based poses difficult can still reap the benefits safely and effectively.

Chair yoga is a testament to yoga's adaptability. It demonstrates that with innovation, yoga's benefits can be accessible to everyone. Remember, it's not about mastering advanced poses but about embracing the journey and the benefits each pose offers your body and mind.

Picture the principles of yoga—concentrate on breathing, a union of mind and body, and poses to enhance flexibility, strength, and inner peace. Now, envision practicing these principles with the aid of a chair. That's chair yoga, in essence. It doesn't dull yoga's effectiveness but makes it more inclusive.

By utilizing a chair as an extension of your body, chair yoga ensures that individuals, especially seniors or those with mobility concerns, can engage in this enriching practice. The chair becomes integral to the yoga session, facilitating balance, deepening stretches, and providing support during challenging poses. At its essence, chair yoga, like all forms of yoga, seeks to establish harmony between mind and body. By adapting poses for accessibility, it offers a gentler approach, making yoga's myriad benefits accessible to those with limited mobility.

**What's so good about Chair Yoga?**

It's a Great use of space: If you have one room and a chair, that's all you need to make your own yoga studio.

Proper posture is crucial, and the chair serves as a support system to achieve correct alignment without straining the body. If, like me, you find maintaining balance a task in traditional yoga poses, the chair provides essential support, allowing us to stretch further and improving the workout.

Chair yoga gently stretches and strengthens muscle groups, improving flexibility. Like traditional yoga, chair yoga emphasizes mindfulness and deep breathing, reducing stress, calming the mind, and enhancing focus. In our fast-paced world, carving out time for chair yoga can be a peaceful oasis, rejuvenating both body and mind. In a rapidly moving world, chair yoga offers a reprieve by emphasizing slow movements and deliberate thinking. Each pose and deep breath offers a moment of appreciation. Despite being seated, chair yoga provides surprising flexibility and cardiovascular benefits with regular practice. From twists to stretches, each pose aims to maintain suppleness and agility, while deep breathing and sustained poses ensure a steady workout for the heart. Over time, this can lead to improved circulation, reduced risk of cardiovascular diseases, and overall better heart health.

Chair yoga transcends mere yoga performed on a chair; it's a testament to yoga's adaptability and its ability to evolve to meet our needs. Whether it's the challenges of aging, space constraints, or physical limitations, chair yoga provides a perfect solution for regaining vitality. Traditional yoga has a rich history spanning hundreds of years. While some may view it through the lens of Eastern philosophy, yoga's benefits have transcended cultural boundaries and resonated globally. In ancient India, yoga became a versatile discipline promoting physical, mental, and emotional well-being. Yoga improves flexibility, strength, and posture. It fosters mindfulness, stress reduction, and increased focus, which are highly sought after in today's fast-paced world. It's important to note that embracing yoga doesn't require adopting an Eastern worldview. Instead, it's a practical approach to self-care, promoting physical health and mental clarity.

**After Exercise, you must rest and recover**

Let's remember that exercise is just one piece of the puzzle. When we engage in any workout, we must prioritize rest and recovery. Sleep is crucial for our bodies when they repair, restore, and rejuvenate. Quality sleep is as essential as the air we breathe. Getting a good night's sleep, ranging from 7 to 9 hours after a workout, is vital. It ensures muscle recovery, mental rejuvenation, and overall well-being. In essence, sleep ensures we reap the benefits of exercise. This is where chair yoga works; The calming sequences, synchronized breathing, and gentle stretches prepare you for deep, restful sleep. They ease tension, calm racing thoughts, and create a serene environment conducive to sleep. But it's not just about falling asleep—it's about the depth of that slumber. With its emphasis on relaxation and mindfulness, chair yoga helps ensure that sleep is deep and uninterrupted once embraced. The mind learns to let go, releasing its grip on anxieties and worries, allowing the body to sink into a state of restorative rest.

In chair yoga, we integrate relaxation techniques that help reduce the stress hormone cortisol, ultimately providing tranquility and rejuvenation. As we stretch and breathe slowly, we release anxieties and stress, simplifying stress management with practice. Chronic or acute pain can hinder daily activities, but chair yoga emerges as an effective form of pain management. Through gentle stretches targeting pain points and deep breathing techniques, tension is eased, and relief is provided. Chair yoga also offers a haven for those grappling with high blood pressure. Synchronized breathwork encourages oxygen flow, promoting vascular health and calming the body amidst blood pressure fluctuations.

Furthermore, chair yoga strengthens the core—the central part of the body that supports and balances the rest. Various poses target the core, enhancing muscles and flexibility and ensuring a strong, supportive core, which is particularly beneficial for alleviating common back pain. Additionally, chair yoga sequences help maintain spine flexibility, strength, and health, offering relief from issues like herniated discs and stiffness. Even past injuries, with their subtle imprints, can be addressed through chair yoga's gentle stretches, promoting better blood flow, easing tension, and overall well-being. Lastly, chair yoga takes a holistic approach to respiratory health by emphasizing deep, diaphragmatic breathing, enhancing lung capacity, and strengthening respiratory muscles to ensure robust lung function, which is particularly beneficial for individuals with respiratory issues like asthma.

Chair yoga is holistic, all about a spirited mindset, and the benefits can be inspirational. Keep this in mind to improve your fitness journey.

# Prepare Yourself

"Growing old is mandatory; growing up is optional." – Chili Davis

Embracing Chair Yoga: Preparing for a Fulfilling Journey.

Get ready to embark on a journey to a healthier mind and body – and yes, it's going to be testing at first, But before we dive in headfirst, let's take a moment to get organized. Trust me, a little prep work now will make all the difference down the road.

First things first: let's talk about your chair for yoga. It's not just about comfort; it's about stability and support. Your chair will be your trusty companion throughout your new exercise routine, so picking the right one is key. Look for a chair with a straight back, no arms, and sturdy legs with no wheels.

When you're seated, both feet should comfortably touch the floor, and keep the padding minimal – you don't want to sink too deep! Remember, your chair is your anchor for confident exploration of stretches and poses, so choose wisely and get ready to test it.

Let's talk about clothing. While it might seem like a small detail, what you wear can totally make or break your moves. Since you're chilling at home, forget about fashion rules and focus on what helps you move best. Think flexible, breathable threads that let you bust out those killer stretches without any hold-ups. And as for footwear, why not ditch the shoes and go barefoot? It'll make you feel super connected to the ground as you flow through your poses; if that doesn't suit you, light footwear will work; it is not too loose, and you don't want them slipping off during stretches.

Now, let's chat about your "yoga room" – pick a spot that's zen and free from distractions. You'll want plenty of space to stretch out, so clear the floor of any obstacles that might trip you up.

Lastly, let's get your mind in the game! Take a second to chill out, get into the zone, and give yourself permission to move at your own pace. When you've got the right chair, the perfect outfit, and a sweet setup, you're all set for an epic chair yoga session that's effective and worthwhile.

Here are some pointers to make sure you nail it safely and effectively.

First things first, let's talk stretching – it's all about finding that sweet spot between effort and ease. You want to feel the stretch, but none of that discomfort, no bouncing around like a maniac – that's a one-way ticket to injury.

Next up, let's master that form and technique – we're talking precision here. Warming up those muscles is crucial to avoid injuries and get the most out of your session. Trust me; gentle movements aren't just for show – they prime your body and mind for greatness.

And speaking of greatness, alignment is key. Feet flat, back straight, and shoulders chilled – it's like setting the stage for a killer performance every time. Plus, paying attention to your form now means you'll be reaping the benefits for years to come.

Now, Chair Yoga isn't a race – it's a journey. So take it slow, embrace those fluid movements, and listen to what your body's telling you. And hey, as you progress, you're gonna start feeling like a superhero – stronger, more flexible, unstoppable.

Oh, and let's not forget about hydration and nutrition – they're like the secret sauce to your fitness success! Stay tuned for more juicy tips on that in our next session. But for now, let's dive headfirst into our first routine, armed with these pointers for a safe and kickass Chair Yoga session.

## Quick Warm-Up Exercises

It's time to bring positivity and energy into our day with awesome chair yoga stretches. Get ready to light up your space and get your body moving with this beginner-friendly routine. It's easy and fun – the perfect way to get your body limbered up and feeling good.

## First Warm-up Routine

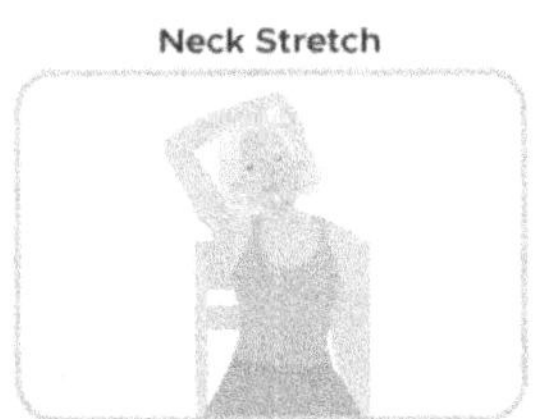



**Neck Stretches:** Start off with some Gentle head Tilts. Keep that back nice and straight, and gently place your left hand on the right side of your head. Take a deep breath in through your nose as you tilt your head towards your left shoulder, then exhale as you hold the pose. Feel that stretch, and hold it for a couple of breaths. Then, go back to the center and repeat – Switch it up to the other side and give it another go. Inhale, tilt, exhale – Do this four times

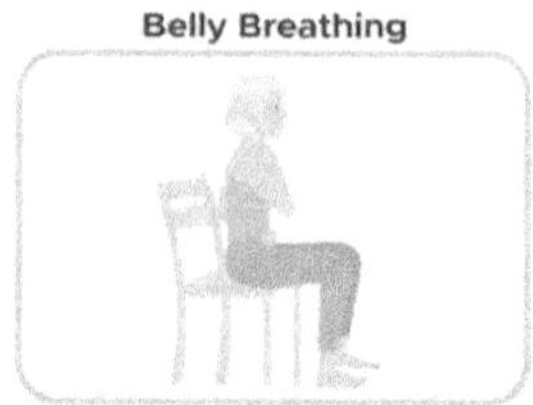

Belly Breathing

**Deep Breathing:** Now, let's dive into some Deep Breathing. Sit tall in your chair, close those eyes, and take a big, deep breath through your nose. Exhale slowly through your mouth – let it all out nice and slow. Focus on your breath, feeling it calm your mind and set you for the session ahead, in and out, in and out. Do this ten times.

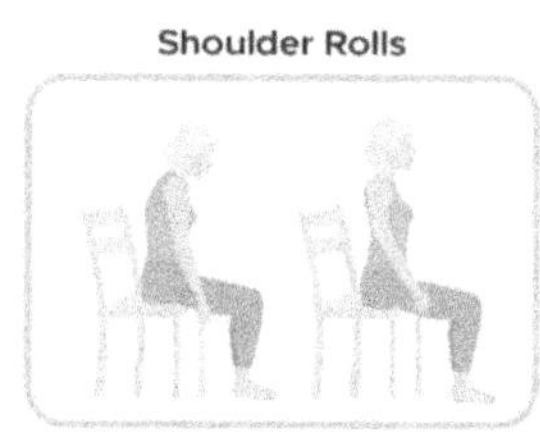

Shoulder Rolls

Shoulder Rolls: Inhale as you lift them up and roll them forward, then exhale as you roll them back and down. Feel that tension melt away with each roll. Let's do that a few times, then switch it up – inhale as you lift them up and roll them backward, then exhale as you drop them down and roll them forward. Keep those breaths flowing and stay mindful of your every move – you're doing amazing! Do these six times.

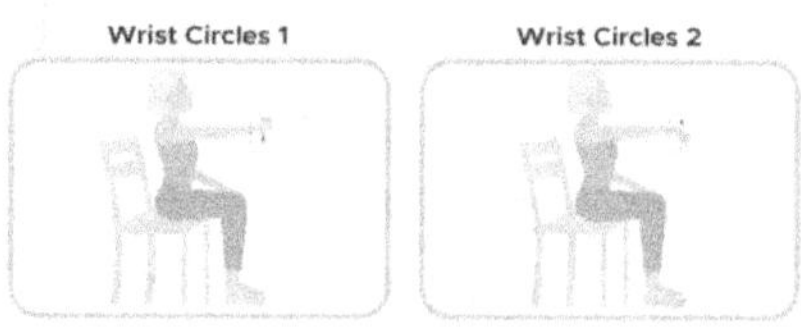

Wrist Circles 1          Wrist Circles 2

**Wrist Rotation:** As you inhale, extend your arms in front of you with palms facing down. Begin gently rotating the wrists in a clockwise direction as you exhale. Count: Two, Three, Four, Five. Pause, inhale, and rotate in the opposite direction as you exhale. Count: Two, Three, Four, Five. Lower your arms, inhale slowly, hold, then exhale.

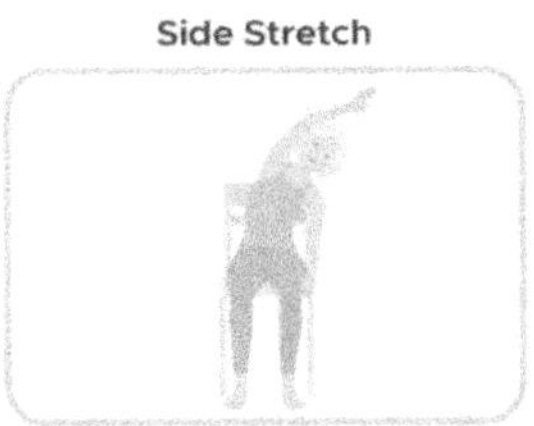
Side Stretch

**Gentle Side Stretching:** Stretch your arms overhead while inhaling through your nose. Breathe out and lean to the right side for a gentle stretch. Return to the center while inhaling, then lean to the left while exhaling. Concentrate on feeling the stretch in your sides and lean into it, but avoid overstretching. Repeat this movement six times for each side.

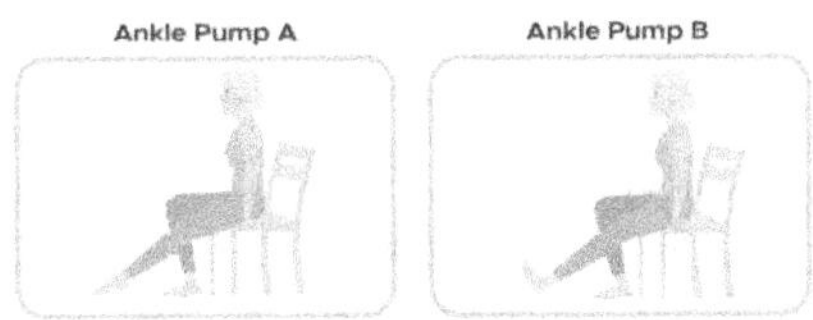
Ankle Pump A          Ankle Pump B

**Ankle Pumps:** Keep your feet flat by lifting your heels while keeping your toes on the floor. Lower the heels back down, then lift the toes. Repeat this movement five times. You can lift both heels at the same time or alternate between them.

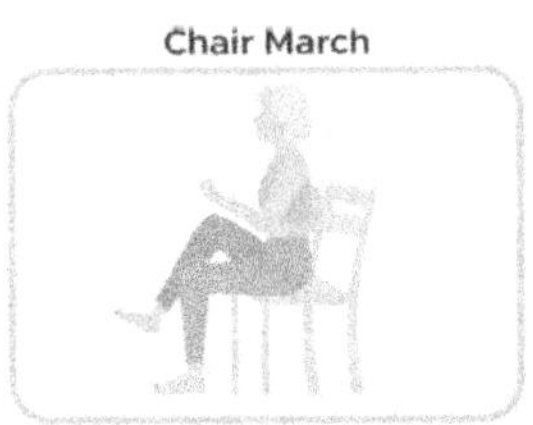
Chair March

**Chair March** (can also be done standing next to your chair): Sit straight with your feet on the floor and your arms bent at the elbows. Begin by lifting your right foot and left arm up while pushing your right arm back. Transition to lifting your left arm and right foot as if you were marching. Keep up this motion for 2 to 3 minutes at a moderate pace.

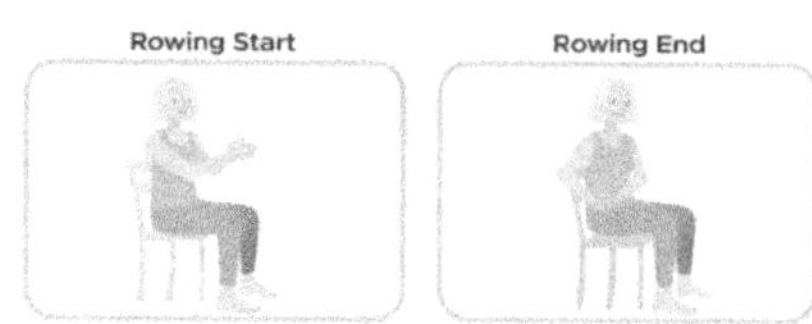


**Seated Rows:** Alright, Let's dive into some seated rowing to fire up those muscles and get that heart pumpin'! Sit forward in your chair, hands clasped together, and stretch 'em out to your left side. Now, let's row that imaginary boat with some medium-speed pulls from front to back – feel that burn! With four reps on each side, switch it up to the right side and repeat. We're doing this whole sequence four times – let's crush it!

These quick warm-up exercises are more than just stretches – they're your secret weapon for muscle relaxation, increased circulation, and getting your body revved up for your daily grind. Plus, they're the perfect way to kickstart your morning and set the tone for a killer day ahead!

So there you have it, folks – a kickass chair yoga warmup routine to kickstart your day with a bang! Keep that energy high.

## Dietary Tips

As people cross the threshold of 60, their nutritional needs evolve, necessitating a more mindful approach to diet and hydration to support sustained health and vitality. One of the most important dietary tips for this age group is reducing junk food intake significantly.

Processed foods high in unhealthy fats, sugars, and sodium can exacerbate age-related health issues such as heart disease, type 2 diabetes, and hypertension. Instead, individuals over 60 should prioritize a diet rich in whole foods, including plenty of fruits, vegetables, lean proteins, whole grains, and healthy fats like those found in avocados, nuts, and olive oil.

Proper hydration is crucial, as the body's ability to conserve water diminishes with age. Drinking adequate amounts of water daily supports metabolism, aids in digestion, and helps maintain energy levels. Hydration becomes even more critical during exercise, which is essential for maintaining muscle mass and overall fitness.

Sweating leads to the loss of water and essential electrolytes, such as sodium, potassium, and magnesium, which are vital for muscle function and preventing cramps. To stay well-hydrated and maintain electrolyte balance, it is advisable to drink water regularly and consume electrolyte-rich foods like bananas, oranges, spinach, and yogurt. Sometimes, an electrolyte-replenishing sports drink may be beneficial, particularly during prolonged or intense physical activity. By cutting down on junk food, ensuring proper hydration, and maintaining electrolyte levels during exercise, individuals over 60 can effectively support their health and fitness, paving the way for a more energetic and vibrant life.

So, let's make hydration and nutrition a priority, folks! Drink up, fuel up, and let's crush those workouts together.

To fuel our bodies for those killer workouts, we've gotta get our nutrition game on point! As we grow older, our bodies need different things to keep us going strong, which is why a balanced diet packed with all the good stuff is crucial.

Let's break it down: first up, we've got protein – the building blocks for those strong muscles. Think lean options like chicken, fish, tofu, and beans to give your body what it needs to repair and grow.

Next, load up on fruits and veggies – they're like nature's multivitamin, packed with all the good stuff to keep inflammation at bay and boost overall health.

Don't forget about whole grains – they're the fuel that keeps your energy levels steady and your digestion on point. Brown rice, quinoa, and whole wheat bread are where it's at!

And hey, dairy or dairy alternatives? They're not just for kids! Low-fat options are loaded with calcium and vitamin D to keep those bones nice and strong as we age.

Now, let's talk about fats – the good kind, that is! Avocados, nuts, seeds, and olive oil are your go-tos for heart health and long-lasting energy.

But hold up – not all foods are created equal. Skip the sugary snacks, processed foods, and greasy fries. They might give you a quick energy boost but leave you feeling sluggish and inflamed in the long run.

Let's talk about making smart choices when it comes to our eats – especially as we get older and wiser. Here are some key tips to keep in mind, especially for those of us who are rocking the 60-plus club!

First up, let's cut back on the sugary and processed stuff. Those sneaky snacks and drinks might give you a quick buzz, but they'll leave you crashing hard later on. Plus, processed foods are often loaded with unhealthy fats and way too much sodium – not cool!

Speaking of sodium, let's keep an eye on that salt intake. Too much can wreak havoc on your blood pressure, which ain't great for your heart health. So, go easy on the salty stuff, and your ticker will thank you!

And don't even get me started on trans fats. These bad boys are hiding out in all sorts of processed and fried foods, causing inflammation and upping your risk of heart issues. Let's steer clear of those greasy traps, shall we?

By focusing on nutrient-packed foods and avoiding the not-so-healthy options, we're setting ourselves up for success—both in our workouts and in life. So, let's fuel our bodies right, crush those workouts, and keep our immune systems strong and resilient. We've got this!

Opt for nutrient-dense foods that are packed with essential vitamins, minerals, and antioxidants – they're like the superheroes of your diet, supporting your exercise routine and overall well-being. These powerhouse foods help you maintain energy levels and keep those muscles in tip-top shape.

By making smart dietary choices and putting these nutrient-rich foods at the top of your grocery list, you're setting yourself up for a lifetime of health and vitality. But hey, it's always a good idea to chat with your healthcare provider before making any big changes to your diet, especially if you've got medical conditions or are taking medications. Your doc can give you personalized advice that's tailored to your unique needs and goals.

Now, let's talk about some amazing foods that are famous for their anti-inflammatory superpowers. These tasty treats can work wonders for your health, so why not add a few to your daily meals?

First up, we've got berries – think blueberries, strawberries, raspberries, and blackberries. They're bursting with antioxidants called anthocyanins, which are like little inflammation-fighting ninjas.

Next, let's explore fatty fish like salmon, mackerel, sardines, and herring. These ocean goodies are rich in omega-3 fatty acids, which are known for their inflammation-reducing properties.

Remember broccoli—this green machine is packed with sulforaphane, an antioxidant that fights inflammation and promotes overall health.

Last but not least, we have peppers—both bell peppers and chili peppers. They're loaded with quercetin, synaptic acid, and ferulic acid, all of which are effective in fighting inflammation.

# Fitness Test

This book is designed to increase your fitness and hopefully improve your life; firstly, you need to know how fit you are now so you can compare the you now to the you afterwards.

Firstly we all know that Individuality is a major factor when it comes to fitness. Age, lifestyle, health conditions, and other variables all contribute to shaping one's fitness level at any given age, including 60. However, this doesn't mean that it's not important to strive for optimal fitness. In fact, as we age, it becomes increasingly crucial to maintain an active and healthy lifestyle.

Older adults have a wide range of fitness levels. While some may have difficulty with activities such as climbing stairs, others may be able to accomplish feats like running marathons. So, what level of fitness should you aim for at 60? We don't want to compare you to anyone else. We want to improve what you already have.

There are various guidelines and fitness assessments that can help you gauge your fitness level. These results can provide a starting point, but it's crucial to seek guidance from your physician for a comprehensive evaluation. This step ensures your safety and reassures you that you're on the right track.

Take the following five tests and note your results. Then, after you've completed the 28-day program, re-test and look at how much you have improved.

## The 6-minute walk test

The 6-minute walk test is a simple and quick exercise that can help assess your aerobic capacity. The goal is to walk as far as possible on a flat and hard surface in six minutes, using only a stopwatch.

Simply count the distance or measure the steps and see if you improve after the 28-day routine.

If you're not sure how to measure the distance you've walked, you can use a step counter, such as a Fitbit or pedometer. You can also mark a starting and ending point and count the number of back-and-forth trips you make between them.

The best way to improve your endurance is to walk regularly, which can be enjoyable for many people. Aim to take a walk every day until it becomes habitual. If you're ready to take it up a notch, try jogging, running, swimming, or other forms of aerobic exercise. Even if you have to shorten your sessions to fit them into your daily routine, consistency is key.

## Chair Stand Test

The Chair Stand is a fitness test designed to measure lower body strength. All you need to conduct it are a stable chair and a stopwatch.

To start, ensure that the chair is stable and place it against a wall. Sit in the middle with your feet shoulder-width apart and cross your arms at the wrists, holding them to your chest. From the sitting position, stand up completely and then sit back down again. Repeat this as many times as possible in 30 seconds.

How did you do? Simply mark the results and see if you beat it after the 28-day routine.

## Biceps Curl

The Biceps Curl is a fitness test that assesses upper body strength and endurance. To perform it, you'll need a stopwatch and a dumbbell. Women should use a 5 lb (2.27 kg) weight, while men should use an 8 lb (3.63 kg) weight.

Begin by sitting on a chair and holding the weight in your hand with your palm facing towards you. Keep your arm close to your body, ensuring that only the lower part of your arm is moving. Then, bend your arm fully and straighten out your elbow. The objective is to complete as many bicep curls as possible within 30 seconds.

After completing the test, mark your results and strive to beat them after following a 28-day routine.

Research suggests that nutrition is crucial in both muscle-building and weight loss. Therefore, please check out our guide for more information on nutrition for older adults. With the right combination of weight training and nutrition, you will see a significant improvement in your muscle strength and firmness over time.

## Single Stance Test

The Single Stance Test is a straightforward yet effective way to measure your static and dynamic balance. To perform the test, you only need a stopwatch.

To begin the test, stand on one leg while placing your hands on your hips. Start the timer as soon as your foot is bent at the knee. Stop the timer when your foot touches the ground again or when you move your hands from your hips.

The results of the test are easy to interpret. If you are over 60 years old and can stand for more than five seconds, you should be satisfied with your balance.

Maintaining good balance is essential for staying healthy and independent. To improve your balance, you can try incorporating yoga, tai-chi, or even dance lessons into your weekly exercise routine. These activities can help reduce your risk of falling and set you up for successful aging.

## Chair sit and reach

The Chair Sit and Reach Test is a great way to measure your flexibility. To perform this test, you will need a ruler, a chair, and someone to assist you in measuring the results.

To begin, sit on the edge of a chair with one foot firmly on the ground. Straighten your other leg and place your heel on the ground.

Next, place your hands on top of each other and take a deep breath. As you exhale, slowly reach forward towards your toes, keeping your knee straight. Be sure to avoid any sudden movements, bouncing, or stretching to the point of pain.

Finally, have your partner measure the distance between the tips of your fingertips and toes. If you can touch your toes, your score is zero. If you cannot reach them (a negative score) or your fingertips overlap with your toes (a positive score), measure the difference.

After completing the test, mark your results and strive to beat them after following a 28-day routine.

# Breathing



"Life is like a roll of toilet paper. The closer you get to the end, the faster it goes." – Anonymous.

Welcome to a short chapter dedicated to the profound journey of reconnecting with your body through mindful breathing. In our fast-paced world, it's easy to become disconnected from the intricate workings of our physical selves. Yet, as we age, the importance of fostering a deep and meaningful connection with our bodies becomes increasingly apparent.

For many individuals over 60, the journey of aging can bring about a myriad of changes, both physically and emotionally. Our bodies may not move as they once did, and we may face new challenges and limitations. However, within these changes lies an opportunity for growth, self-discovery, and profound connection.

Connecting with our bodies goes beyond mere physicality; it encompasses a holistic understanding of ourselves—mind, body, and spirit. It's about cultivating awareness, acceptance, and appreciation for the vessel that carries us through life's journey.

## Honoring Your Body's Wisdom

As we age, our bodies accumulate a wealth of wisdom born from years of experience and resilience. Each wrinkle, scar, and ache tells a story—a testament to our journey. Yet, in our youth-obsessed culture, it's easy to overlook the beauty and wisdom inherent in aging.

Connecting with your body means honoring and respecting the wisdom it holds. It's about listening to its cues, acknowledging its needs, and treating it with the love and care it deserves. By embracing a mindset of self-compassion and acceptance, we can cultivate a deeper sense of connection with our bodies, fostering a relationship built on trust and understanding.

## Cultivating Movement as Medicine

Movement is not just about physical fitness; it's a form of self-expression, a celebration of what our bodies are capable of achieving. For those over 60, staying active becomes increasingly important for maintaining physical health and nurturing our connection with our bodies.

Incorporating gentle movement practices such as yoga, tai chi, or walking can be transformative, allowing us to reconnect with our bodies in a gentle and compassionate way. These practices encourage us to move with intention and save the sensation of each breath, stretch, and step. They invite us to inhabit our bodies fully, embracing their inherent strength, flexibility, and resilience.

Think of the brain as a plant that requires regular nourishment to thrive. Just like plants need water to flourish, our brains rely on a steady blood supply for optimal function. Unfortunately, blood flow to the brain decreases as we age, affecting cognitive processes. This decline in resources doesn't mean occasional forgetfulness is inevitable but rather signifies the brain's adaptation to changing circumstances.

Achieving body harmony through breath is essential as we age, especially considering the changes our brains undergo, affecting cognitive functions like memory and processing speed. Chair yoga, when combined with proper breathing techniques, becomes a powerful tool for maintaining mental acuity by enhancing blood flow. In chair yoga workouts, breathing plays a central role; our lungs and brains work together during breathing, and mastering an efficient technique can significantly improve overall health outcomes.

Engaging in mindful chair yoga combines breathing, focus, and movement, providing a natural remedy for stress and enhancing mental clarity. Breathing isn't just a passive activity; it actively shapes our mental and emotional states. When synchronized with purposeful chair yoga movements, breathing helps disperse stress and boosts mental acuity.

Mindfulness is key to unlocking the full benefits of breathwork. In chair yoga, being mindful of breathwork is akin to appreciating a beautiful piece of music and understanding each note's role in the composition. This transforms chair yoga into a profound practice as you become an observer of your own breath, fostering inner peace and well-being.

A couple of basic Breathwork Techniques

Breathing is not just about staying alive—it has the power to rejuvenate our bodies and minds from within. If you are used to concluding your day with a rush of random screen time or busy tasks, imagine ending it with a quiet moment of mindful breathing. Just a few minutes dedicated to breathing can realign your mind and body. It's a simple practice that can enhance sleep quality and life quality. And it's not limited to bedtime.

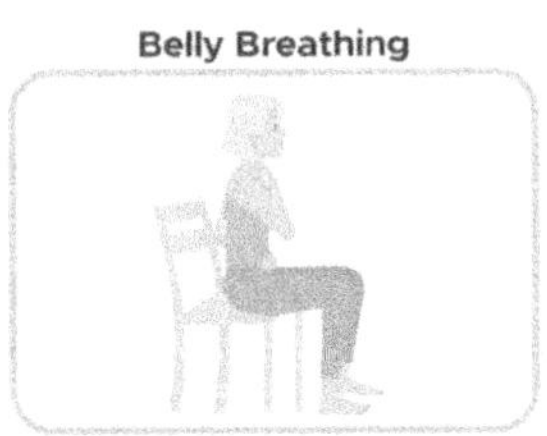


Breathing (Diaphragmatic Breathing):

Belly breathing is a fantastic introduction to conscious breathing. Especially for beginners. Focusing on activating the diaphragm, a vital muscle beneath the lungs. Begin by sitting comfortably with a straight back in a chair. Place a hand on your chest and a hand on your belly.

Inhale deeply through your nose, letting your belly expand while keeping your chest still. Hold for a moment, then exhale slowly through your mouth, sucking your belly inward. Repeat this process for a few minutes, closely observing the rise and fall of your belly.

Breath of the Ocean:

This breathing exercise adds a layer of complexity by engaging the throat, which forms a soothing, meditative quality that goes perfectly with the gentle movements of chair yoga. Sit straight in your chair with relaxed shoulders. Slowly inhale through your nose, and as you exhale, gently constrict the back of your throat, creating a soft sound akin to fogging a pane of glass. Aim to maintain this gentle sound throughout both inhalation and exhalation. Repeat this exercise for a few minutes, and as you do, try to clear and relax your mind. It's a fantastic way to remove the day's stresses and be mindful of your body and health.

Try to get into the habit of taking a few quiet minutes to breathe like this every day, and watch it improve your mental and physical health.

# How to get Flexible

"The best tunes are played on the oldest fiddles!" - *Ralph Waldo Emerson*

Welcome to the exciting journey of enhancing flexibility! In this chapter, we'll delve into the world of flexibility training tailored specifically for individuals in their golden years. Flexibility isn't just about touching your toes; it's about maintaining mobility, independence, and overall well-being as we age. Let's explore practical strategies and gentle exercises designed to improve flexibility, reduce stiffness, and promote a greater range of motion.

Understanding Flexibility:

Before we begin the exercises, let's define flexibility. Flexibility refers to the ability of our muscles and joints to move freely through their full range of motion without discomfort or restriction. As we age, factors such as decreased physical activity, loss of muscle mass, and changes in connective tissue can contribute to a decline in flexibility.

However, it's essential to recognize that age does not determine flexibility. With consistent practice and the right approach, individuals of any age can improve their flexibility and enjoy enhanced mobility. Moreover, flexibility training goes beyond physical benefits; it can alleviate stress, improve posture, and enhance overall quality of life.

Benefits of Flexibility Training:

Engaging in regular flexibility exercises offers a multitude of benefits for individuals over 60. Here are some key advantages:

Improved Joint Health: Flexibility exercises help maintain the health of our joints by promoting lubrication and reducing stiffness. This can alleviate discomfort associated with conditions such as arthritis and osteoarthritis, allowing for greater ease of movement.

Enhanced Mobility: By increasing flexibility, we can improve our range of motion and ability to perform daily activities more quickly and efficiently—tasks such as bending, reaching, and turning become more manageable, enhancing overall functionality.

Injury Prevention: Flexible muscles and joints are less prone to injury, as they can withstand sudden movements and exertion better. Incorporating flexibility training into your routine can help prevent falls, strains, and other injuries common among older adults.

Better Posture and Balance: Flexibility exercises target muscles throughout the body, including those responsible for maintaining proper posture and balance. We can improve alignment, stability, and coordination by stretching and lengthening these muscles.

Stress Relief: Flexibility training encourages relaxation and mindfulness, making it an excellent way to alleviate stress and promote mental well-being. Focusing on the present moment during stretching exercises can help us experience a sense of calm and tranquility.

With these benefits in mind, let's dive into a series of gentle yet effective flexibility exercises to support your journey toward improved mobility and well-being. Remember to listen to your body, breathe deeply, and approach each stretch with mindfulness and intention.

Now that we've explored the importance of flexibility and its myriad benefits let's delve into some gentle yet effective exercises specifically designed for individuals over 60. These exercises are safe, accessible, and adaptable to various fitness levels, making them suitable for everyone, regardless of prior experience or mobility limitations. Whether you're looking to improve flexibility for everyday activities or enhance your overall quality of life, these exercises will set you on the path to success. Let's get started with your breathing!

Breath, like the silent conductor of an orchestra, guides every movement in our chair yoga sessions. The rhythm harmonizes our practice, whether we seek to enhance mobility or relieve stress. As we embark on this journey, let us embrace the profound connection between breath and movement that underpins each guided sequence.

Mobility is the cornerstone of well-being and independence, shaping our ability to navigate the world easily and gracefully. Yet, for many, mobility challenges can cast a shadow over daily life, impacting everything from simple tasks to overall quality of life.

It's crucial to recognize that limited mobility is not solely the domain of aging but a complex interplay of various factors. These factors extend beyond age, affecting individuals of all walks of life:

• **Lack of Physical Activity:** Embracing a sedentary lifestyle gradually erodes muscle strength and joint flexibility, rendering routine activities increasingly arduous.

• **Hearing and Eyesight:** Impaired auditory and visual senses diminish spatial awareness, elevating the likelihood of falls and eroding confidence in navigating one's surroundings.

• **Obesity:** Carrying excess weight places undue strain on joints and muscles, exacerbating mobility challenges and heightening the risk of associated health issues.

• **Balance and Coordination Problems:** Challenges in balance or coordination stemming from vertigo, medication side effects, or other health conditions elevate the risk of falls and curtail physical activity.

By understanding these factors and addressing them with purposeful action, we can reclaim our mobility and restore vitality to our lives.

Through mindful chair yoga practice, combined with targeted exercises and lifestyle adjustments, we pave the way for greater freedom of movement and enhanced well-being. Let's embark on this journey together, empowering ourselves to overcome mobility challenges and embrace life with renewed vigor and confidence.

The repercussions of reduced mobility extend far beyond physical limitations, impacting emotional well-being and fostering a sense of dependency and isolation. Chair yoga emerges as a valuable resource in addressing these challenges, offering adaptable exercises tailored to diverse limitations. Whether through gentle stretches or cardiovascular movements, chair yoga promotes physical well-being and enhances confidence, indirectly aiding sensory impairments.

Despite our overall health, aging inevitably brings changes to our joints and ligaments. Over time, these structures undergo alterations, leading to decreased flexibility and occasional discomfort. Without proper care, may become rigid and uncomfortable as the years pass.

For Improved Mobility:

Regular physical activity is crucial for maintaining and improving flexibility in people over 60 because it helps to keep muscles and joints limber, reduce stiffness, and promote ease of movement. Our muscles naturally lose elasticity as we age, and joints can become stiffer due to decreased synovial fluid production, which lubricates the joints. Regular stretching and exercise counteract these effects by promoting blood flow, which delivers essential nutrients to the muscles and joints, keeping them healthy. Additionally, physical activity encourages the production of synovial fluid, helping joints move more smoothly. By staying active, older adults can maintain their range of motion, prevent injuries, and continue performing daily tasks with greater ease and comfort.

Chair Yoga as the Ideal Solution:

Chair yoga is an ideal solution for getting fit and flexible for those over 60 because it offers a gentle, accessible form of exercise that accommodates different levels of mobility and fitness. Unlike traditional yoga, chair yoga allows participants to perform poses while seated or using a chair for support, making it easier for those with balance issues, joint pain, or limited flexibility to engage in physical activity safely.

Chair yoga enhances flexibility by gently stretching muscles and joints without putting excessive strain on the body. It also helps improve strength and balance, crucial for preventing falls and maintaining independence in older adults. Additionally, chair yoga promotes better circulation, reduces stress, and can be easily modified to suit individual needs, making it a versatile and effective way to stay active and healthy.

In the next section, we'll explore some chair yoga exercises to alleviate joint stiffness and enhance mobility.

Let's begin with our primary stretching sequence.

Basic Stretches:

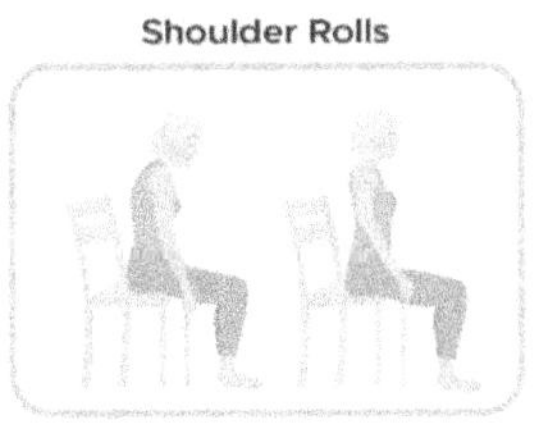


**Shoulder Rolls:** To perform shoulder rolls, start by opening your eyes and inhaling deeply. Lift your shoulders up and roll them forward, then exhale and roll them back and down. Repeat this motion three times, and then reverse it for three times. Remember to stay mindful of your breath throughout the exercise.

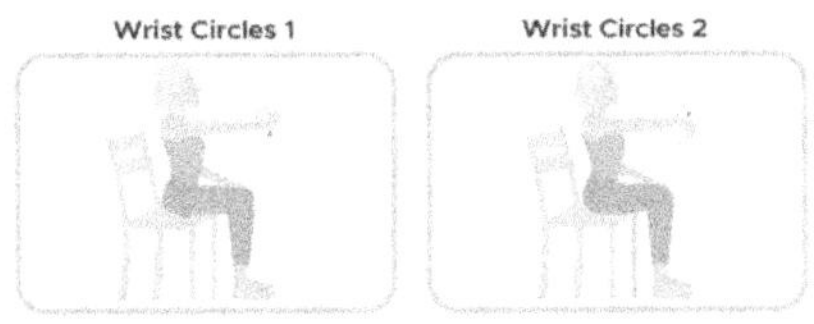

**Wrist Circles:** To perform the Wrist Circles exercise, sit comfortably and extend your arms with palms facing down. Inhale deeply and start rotating your wrists clockwise for five rotations while exhaling. Pause momentarily, inhale, and then rotate your wrists counterclockwise while exhaling. After completing the rotations, lower your arms and take a deep inhale. Hold your breath for a few seconds, and then exhale slowly. This exercise can help to improve flexibility and reduce stiffness in your wrists.

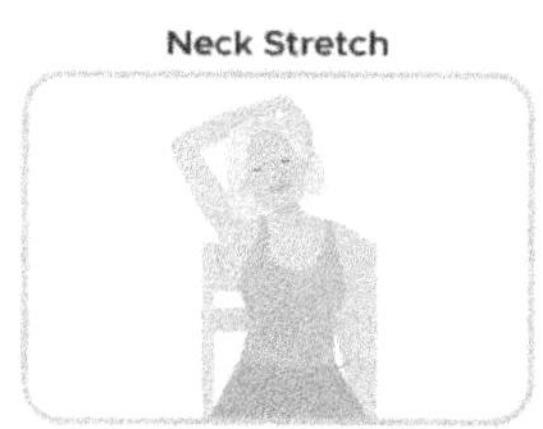


**Neck Stretches:** Keep your back straight, place your hand on the side of your head. Inhale and gently tilt your head towards your shoulder. Hold for two breaths, then switch sides. Repeat once more on each side.

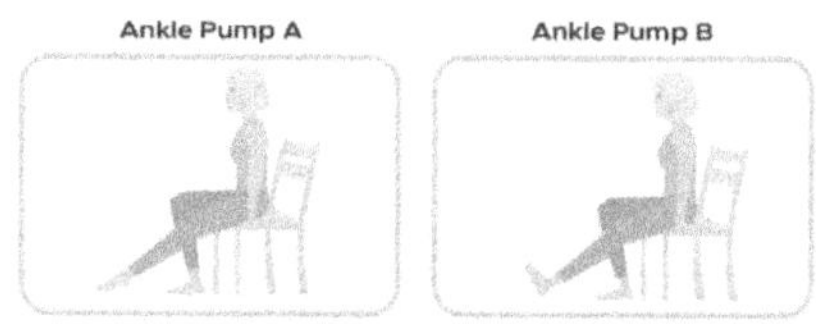


**Ankle Pumps:** Perform the following exercise: First, place your right foot flat on the ground. Then, lift the heel of your left foot slightly while pointing your left foot straight out. After that, lower the left heel while lifting the toes. Repeat this motion 10-20 times. Finally, switch feet and repeat the same steps.

You can also incorporate the Chair March exercise into your warm-ups if desired.

Ok lets begin the main sequence,

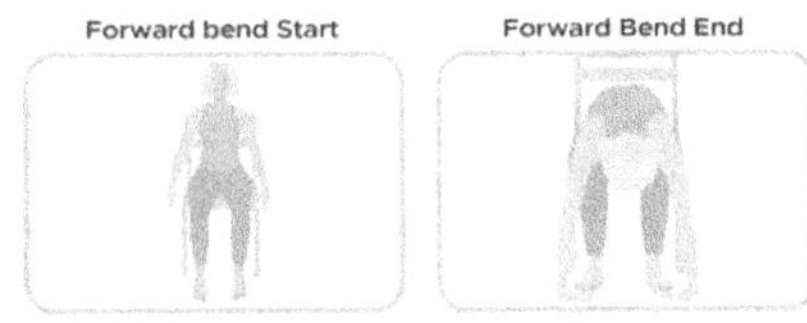



**Forward bend:** The Forward Bend is a yoga pose that targets the spine, hamstrings, and sciatica. Sit up straight, inhale slowly and extend your arms overhead. Exhale and fold from the waist, bringing your hands towards your feet. Hold for ten breaths, keeping your head aligned with your heart. Return to the neutral position.

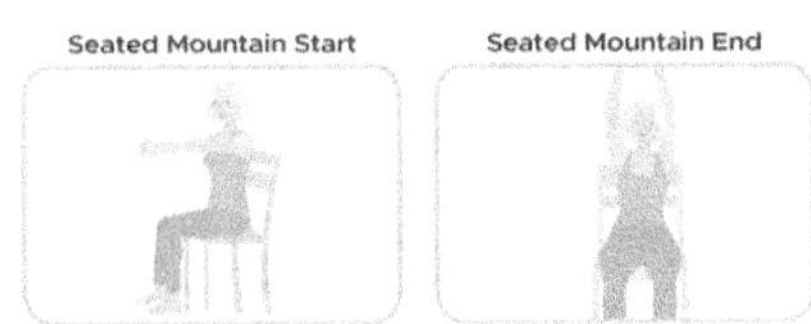



**Seated Mountain:** The seated mountain Pose is a yoga posture that helps cultivate strength and stability in the spine and core. To perform this posture, sit straight with your feet flat on the floor. Inhale deeply as you stretch your arms out, interlocking your fingers and turning your palms outward. Raise your hands above your head with your palms facing the ceiling, aiming to align your head, trunk, and hands. Hold this position for a few breaths before releasing.

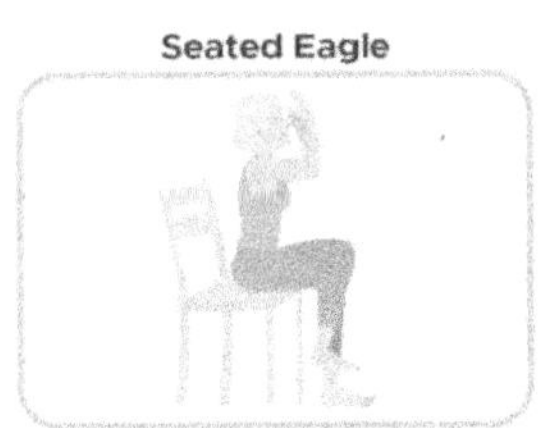



**Seated Eagle Pose:** Cross your right thigh over your left thigh, extend your arms in front, and cross the right arm over the left. Inhale and bend your elbows while bringing your palms together. Hold the pose for a few breaths. Switch sides and repeat with the left thigh over the right. Switch sides: Sit on the edge of the chair and extend your left leg backward. Bend your right knee slightly while keeping your foot on the ground. Inhale slowly through the nose as you raise your arms overhead. Exhale through the mouth as you bend slightly forward while keeping your back straight. Do this six times.

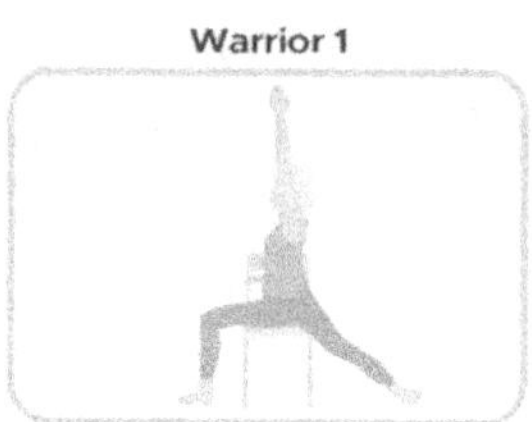



**Warrior Pose:** Here's a posture that can help improve your balance and core strength: Sit sideways on your chair and extend your right leg backwards. Slightly bend your left knee while keeping your foot on the ground. Take a deep breath in through your nose, and as you do so, raise your arms over your head. Exhale slowly through your mouth and bend slightly forward while keeping your back straight. Hold this position for a few breaths."

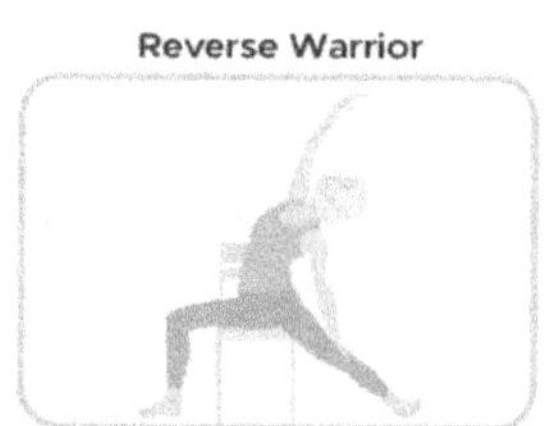



**Reverse Warrior Pose:** this great exercise targets your legs, spine, and core. To get started, sit on the edge of your chair with your right leg extended backward. Place your left hand on your left leg and inhale, looking up as you lift your right arm upwards and backward until your hand touches the top of the chair. Hold this position for a few breaths and then switch sides.

To switch sides, extend your left leg backward and place your right hand on your right leg. Inhale and look up as you lift your left arm upwards and backward until your hand touches the top of the chair. Keep looking up and hold this position briefly before returning to the normal sitting position.

If any of these poses seem too challenging, take a moment to practice diaphragmatic breathing. This therapeutic technique can help prepare your body for the next pose in the sequence.

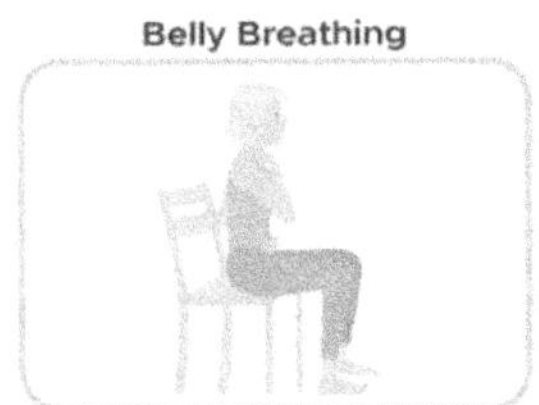


**Diaphram Breathing:** To increase your lung efficiency and reduce stress, sit comfortably and place one hand on your chest and the other on your belly. Breathe in slowly and deeply through your nose, allowing your diaphragm to expand. Exhale completely through your mouth. Repeat this for several breaths.

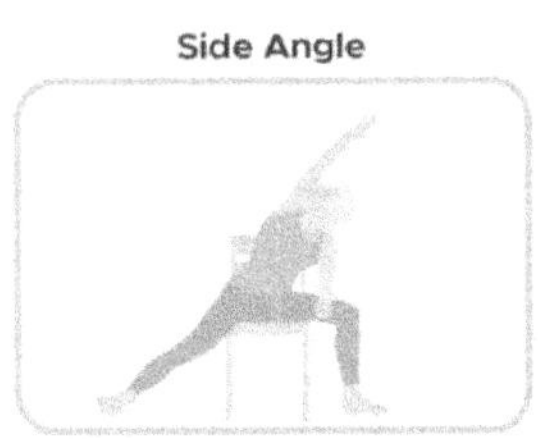


**Side Angle:** Pose is a great stretch for your lower back, legs, and hips. To do this pose, first sit upright with your feet flat on the floor. Place your right hand on your right knee or thigh. Inhale and raise your left arm up towards the ceiling. As you exhale, gently lean to the right, stretching the left side of your body. Hold this position for a few breaths, and then return to your starting position.

Now, repeat on the opposite side. Sit upright with your feet flat on the floor. Place your left hand on your left knee or thigh. Inhale and lift your right arm up towards the ceiling. As you exhale, gently lean to the left, stretching the right side of your body. Hold for a few breaths, then return to your starting position.

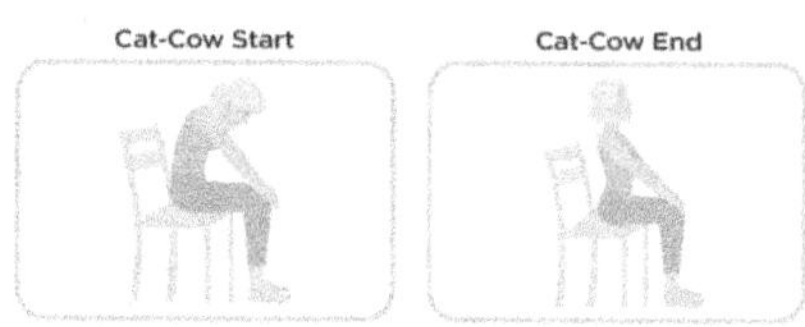


**Cat-Cow Pose** is an excellent exercise for improving balance, posture, and flexibility. Here's how to do it: start by sitting with a straight back and both feet flat on the ground. Place your hands on your knees. As you inhale, arch your back and look up, stretching the front of your neck. As you exhale, round your back, tuck in your chin, and pull the back of your neck. Repeat this movement for several cycles, coordinating your movements with your breaths.

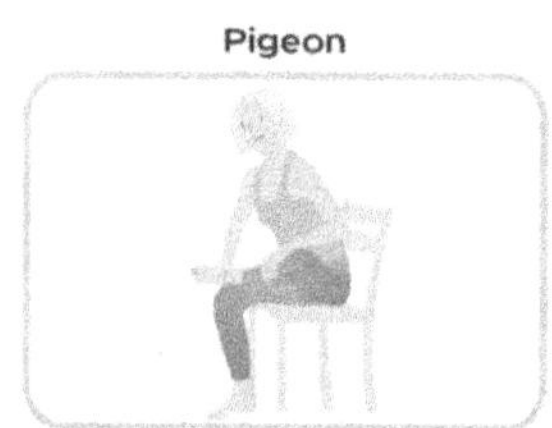


**Pigeon Pose:** Pigeon Pose can help improve mobility and alleviate lower back pain. To do this pose, start by sitting upright with your feet flat on the floor. Lift your right ankle and place it on your left knee, keeping your right knee open. For a deeper stretch, lean slightly forward without rounding your back. Hold this position for several breaths before returning to your normal position.

To stretch the other side of your body, switch sides and repeat the same steps. Sit upright with your feet flat on the floor and lift your left ankle and place it on your right knee. Keep your left knee open and lean slightly forward for a deeper stretch. Hold for several breaths and then return to your normal position.

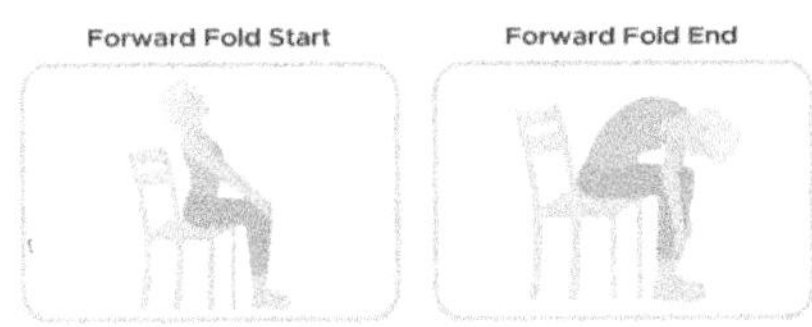


**Forward-Fold:** for Lower Body Flexibility, While seated, place your feet flat on the floor and your hands on your knees. Inhale through your nose and lengthen your spine while looking up. Exhale, hinge at the hips, and fold forward, bringing your chest towards your knees. Allow your hands to grasp the lower legs if possible. Hold for several breaths.

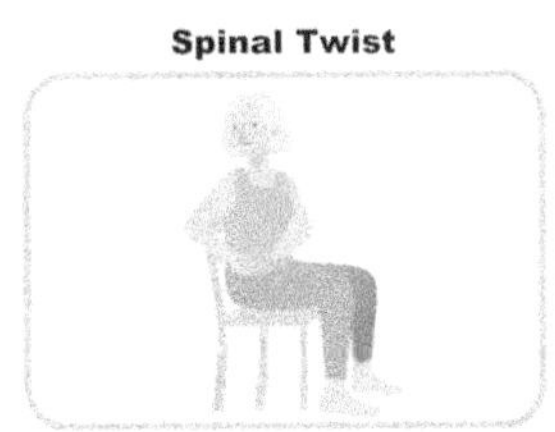


**The Spinal Twist:** The Spinal Twist exercise is highly recommended for enhancing spine flexibility and easing back pain. For performing this exercise, sit upright with your feet placed flat on the floor. Next, place your right hand on your left knee and inhale deeply while lengthening your spine. Then, while exhaling, gently twist towards the left, using your right hand for slight leverage, but be cautious not to twist too far. Hold the position for a few breaths, and then return to a regular position.

Now, switch sides and repeat the exercise. Sit upright with your feet flat on the floor and place your left hand on your right knee. Inhale and lengthen your spine, and then exhale and gently twist to the right, using your left hand for slight leverage. Again, be careful not to twist too far. Hold for several breaths, then return to a normal position.

Breathing: A Refreshing Pause

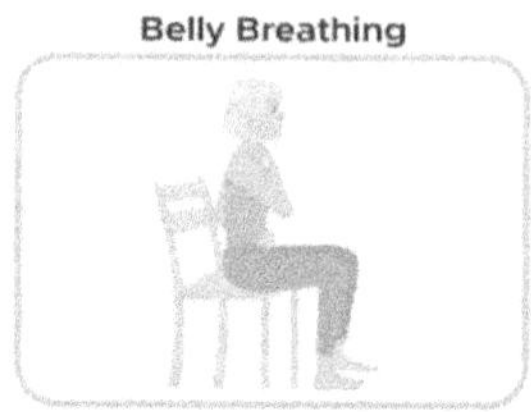


Diaphragmatic breathing is a technique that acts like a reset button for both body and mind. It facilitates smoother transitions between poses and provides a moment to check in with your overall well-being.

To practice diaphragmatic breathing, sit comfortably, place one hand on your chest, and the other on your abdomen. Inhale deeply through the nose, allowing the abdomen to rise as it fills with air, and exhale fully through the mouth. Repeat for several breaths.

Each of these poses offers more than just a physical stretch—they are steps toward better health, improved mobility, and enhanced well-being. By incorporating these poses into your daily routine, you can enhance your mobility, posture, and mental clarity.

## Stiffness

As we age, our joints can become stiff and uncomfortable, limiting our mobility. However, instead of feeling helpless, we can use these limitations to rediscover and expand our abilities. Acceptance is a starting point for innovation and improvement in physical wellness.Effective stretches and well-designed exercises serve as the tools for this expansion. While stretches target specific muscle groups, exercises harmonize different body parts, leading to better balance and functional mobility. The goal isn't just to touch your toes or perform challenging poses but to make daily activities more comfortable, reduce physical stress, and ultimately improve our quality of life.

Stretching becomes more than just a physical movement—it's an exercise in breaking mental barriers as well. Each stretch pushes the limits of what our bodies can do and what we believe is possible. Every slight improvement, every added inch of flexibility, and every newfound ease in movement chips away at the wall of limitation.

"Both acceptance and action are rooted in the present moment, providing an opportunity for growth. Joints lose flexibility due to aging, poor posture, inactivity, being overweight, inflammatory diets, and health conditions. These factors contribute to stiff joints, achy bones, and reduced mobility."So, what's causing the problem? Why do some people's joints move like they're bathed in olive oil while others feel stuck in molasses? Believe it or not, your joints and ligaments have internal clocks. You've probably noticed that your stiffness is worse in the morning. This happens because your body's natural anti-inflammatory substances are at their lowest in the early morning. Wear and tear, leading to discomfort. Poor posture and extra weight can worsen the situation. In the next section, we'll introduce a chair yoga sequence to improve joint flexibility. It's tailored for beginners and those looking to expand their routine.

## Enhancing Flexibility through Exercise

Flexibility is about touching the ground with your hands and expanding your range of possibilities. While it's good to have physical flexibility, you can grab your chair and get comfortable with your new exercise routine. Let's begin with a simple warm-up exercise to increase your flexibility. Breathing exercises are optional but can be included if you'd like.

**Neck Stretch**

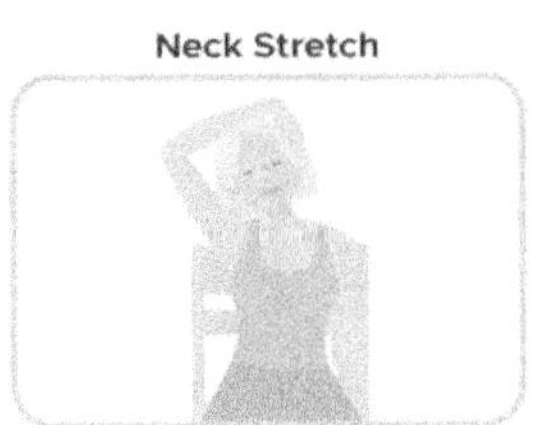

Neck Stretches: Keep your back straight, place your hand on the side of your head. Inhale and gently tilt your head towards your shoulder. Hold for two breaths, then switch sides. Repeat once more on each side.

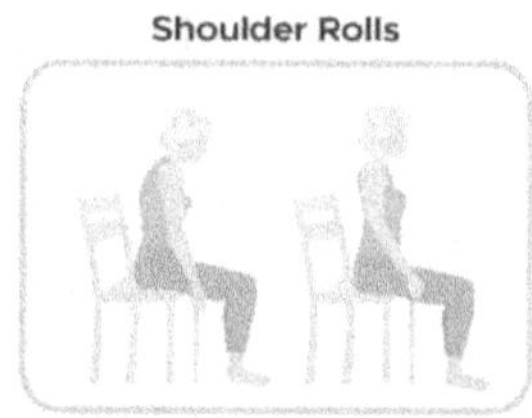



Shoulder Rolls: Close your eyes, inhale, and slowly start rolling your shoulders. Begin by lifting them up and forward and then rolling them back and down while exhaling. Do this three times, then reverse. Inhale, lift up, and roll upward; exhale as you lower down and roll forward. Repeat this five times, and always keep your breathing in mind.

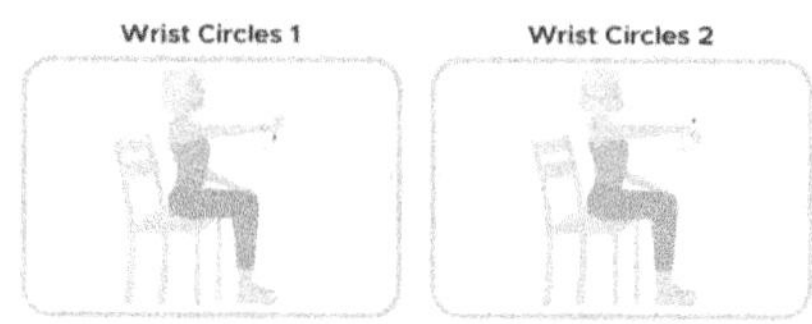



Wrist Circles, To perform wrist circles, extend your arms in front of you with palms facing down while taking a deep breath in. Begin rotating your wrists gently in a clockwise direction for five rotations while exhaling. Count slowly to five as you do this. After five rotations, reverse the movement by inhaling slowly, holding your breath, and then exhaling.

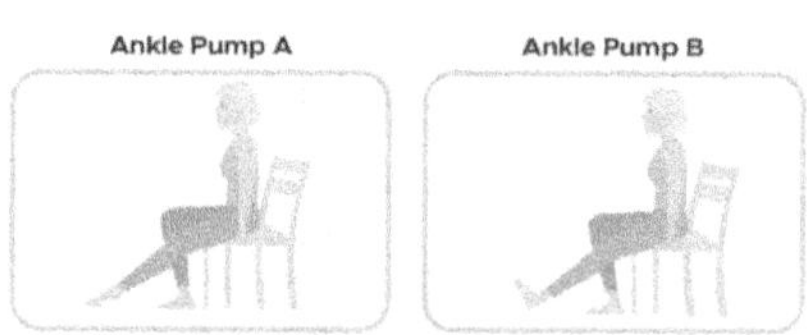



Ankle Pumps: Perform the Ankle Pumps exercise by placing your right foot flat on the ground and lifting your left heel slightly while pointing your left foot straight out. Then, lower the left heel while lifting your toes. Repeat this movement ten times. Next, switch feet and place your left foot flat on the ground. Lift your right heel slightly while pointing your right foot straight out, and lower the right heel while lifting the toes. Repeat this movement ten times as well.

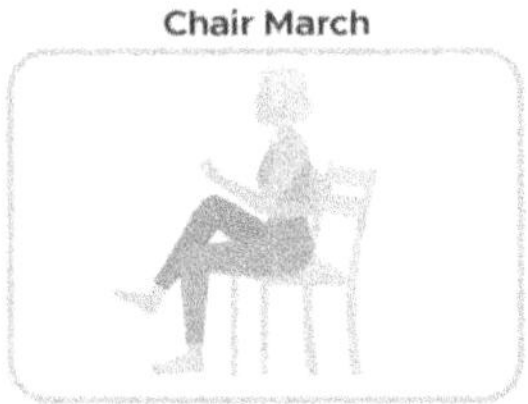

Chair March

To perform Chair March, you can either sit or stand next to your chair. If you choose to sit, keep your feet flat on the floor and your arms bent at the elbows. Begin by lifting your right foot and left arm while pushing your right arm up. Then, switch to the left arm and right foot up, as if you were marching. Keep repeating this motion for 5 minutes at a moderate pace.

Now, onto the main routine. Note: Some exercises may be repeated due to their dual-purpose actions on multiple parts of the body.

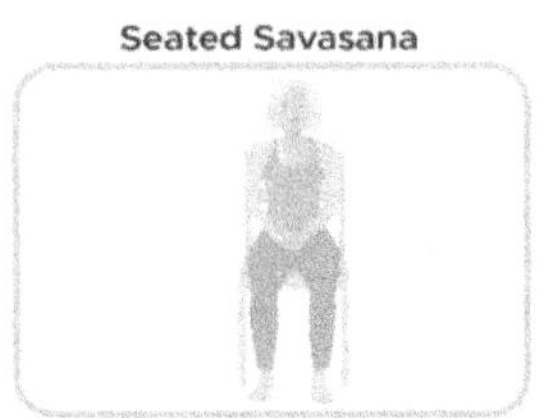

Seated Savasana

Chair Savasana & Relaxation Breathing: To begin, sit comfortably in a chair with your back straight and your feet flat on the ground. Close your eyes and place your hands in your lap. Breathe naturally as you allow your body to relax, starting from the head and moving down the neck, arms, torso, legs, and toes. Stay in this relaxed pose for approximately three minutes. Remember to inhale slowly through the nose, hold briefly, and then exhale through the mouth.

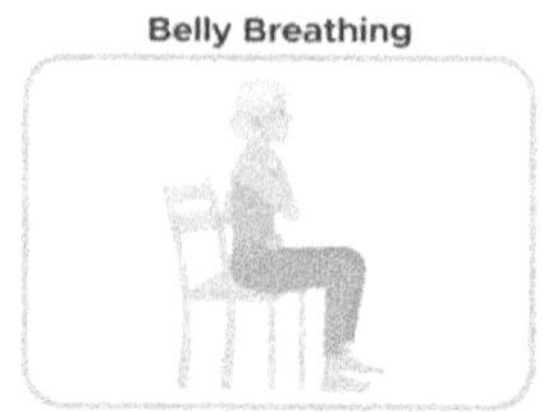



Deep Breathing: To practice deep breathing and relaxation, start by sitting upright. Place one hand on your belly and the other on your chest. Inhale deeply through your nose, slowly filling your abdomen with air. Make sure your chest isn't moving. Then, exhale slowly through your nose. Repeat this cycle ten times. This exercise can help you reduce stress and anxiety, and promote relaxation and calmness.

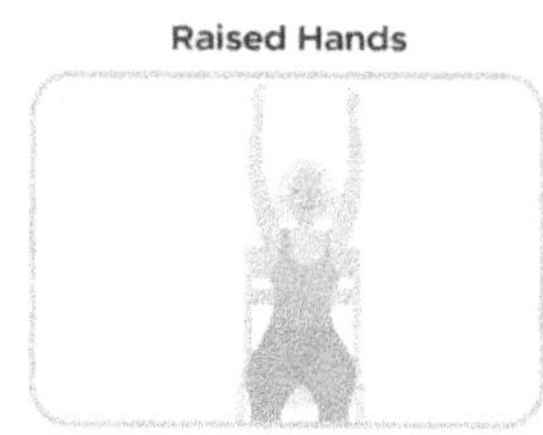



Raised Hands Pose: The Raised Hands Pose is a great way to stretch your arms, shoulders, and upper chest. To do this pose, sit comfortably with your back straight and your feet flat on the floor. Slowly inhale as you raise your arms above your head, aligning them with your ears as much as possible. Make sure your shoulders are relaxed and not hunched. Hold the pose for three to five breaths and then slowly exhale as you lower your hands down to your lap. Arms, Shoulders, Upper Chest: Sit comfortably with your back straight and feet flat on the floor. Inhale slowly as you raise your arms above your head, aligning them with your ears as much as possible. Keep your shoulders relaxed, not hunched. Hold the pose for three to five breaths, then slowly lower your hands down to your lap as you exhale.

Please note the yoga pose below, and remember that it is important to listen to your body and stop if you feel any discomfort. Please do not attempt any pose that is beyond your ability.

## Forward-Fold: Calves, Hamstrings, and Thighs

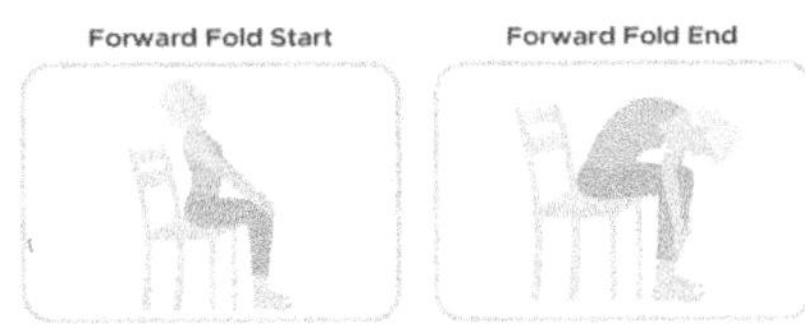


Warning: This pose involves leaning forward. If you feel any discomfort, please return to diaphragmatic breathing as a break.

To perform this pose, sit with your back straight at the edge of the chair, feet flat on the ground. Inhale and bend forward from the waist, stretching the spine and reaching forward towards the floor. Hold onto your ankles with your hands and slide your buttocks forward on the chair to stretch your legs. Hold this pose, inhaling and exhaling slowly for 7-10 breaths. Repeat two times.

Remember to breathe deeply throughout the pose and focus on your breath to help you relax.

The Warrior I and II/Reverse Warrior Pose is a full-body stretch that brings flexibility and a sense of bravery as if preparing for a well-fought battle against stiffness. Although you should aim to transition smoothly from Warrior I to II to Reverse Warrior, you may want to practice each pose separately.

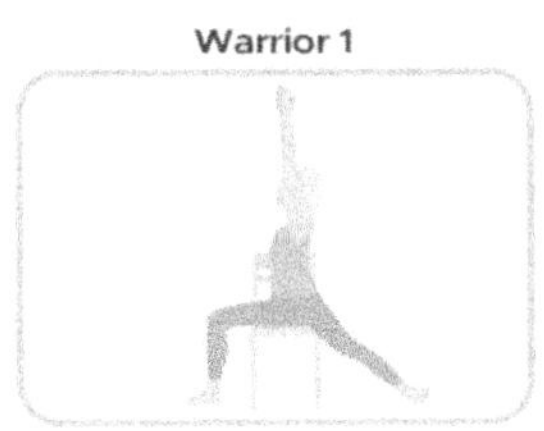


Warrior 1 improves balance, flexibility and strength of the legs, arms, hips, and thighs. To do it, sit sideways on a chair, bring your right leg in front of you, and swing the left leg behind you as you straighten it as much as possible. Keep your torso over the right leg as you raise your arms up to the ceiling while inhaling. The final position should be Warrior I.

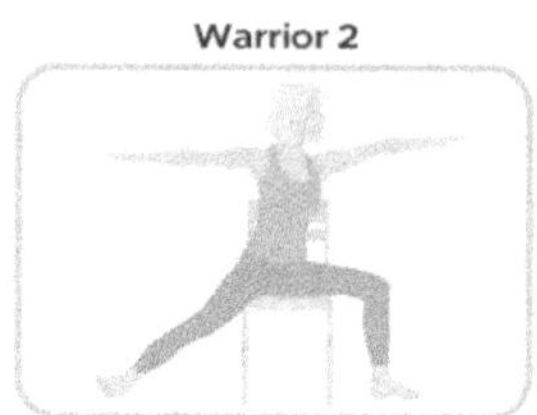


Warrior 2 enhances balance, flexibility, and strength of the legs, arms, and upper body. To do it, turn your torso to face the front of the chair while extending your arms out to the sides, palms facing down. Take deep breaths, inhaling and exhaling three times. The final position should be Warrior II.

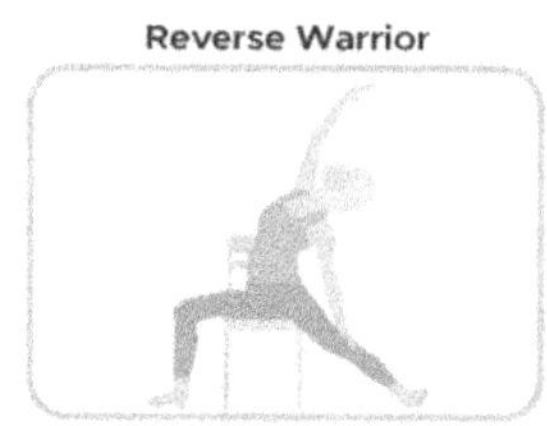


Reverse Warrior promotes flexibility, balance, and strength of the legs, spine, core, and torso. To do it, gently lower your left hand down toward the left foot while lifting your right hand up and bending it slightly over your head, opening up the chest and side of the body. Hold this pose while focusing on deep breaths. The final position should be Reverse Warrior.

Note that the Warrior poses are vigorous, so please take a brief rest before moving on to other exercises, such as forward bends, that can enhance your flexibility.

Single Leg Bend

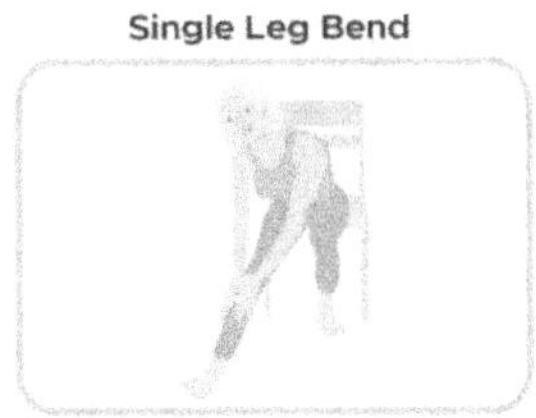

Leg forward bends are great for building strength and increasing flexibility. However, if you have any restrictions related to inversions, modifying this pose and taking a break is recommended. Diaphragmatic breathing is always a safe choice. To perform this pose, start by sitting straight with your feet flat on the ground. Inhale and extend one leg straight in front of you while keeping the other foot flat on the floor. As you exhale, bend forward towards the extended leg and try to touch your toes. Hold for three to five breaths and then repeat with the opposite leg.

Hero

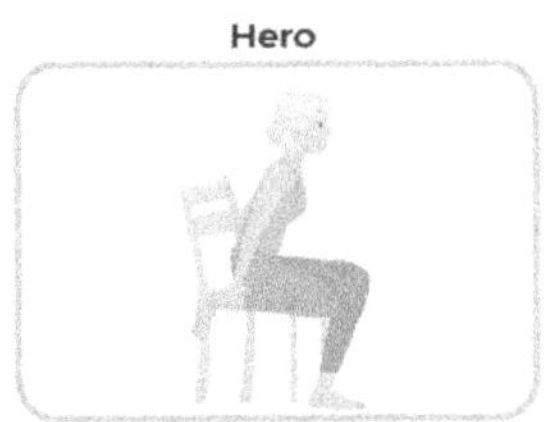

Hero's Pose is a yoga pose that helps to strengthen your quadriceps, knees, ankles, and thighs. To perform this pose, sit comfortably on a chair with your feet flat on the ground. Slide to the front edge of the seat and extend your left leg up, keeping the knee bent. Ensure that your bent knee is pointing downwards and the foot is flat against the side of the chair. Hold this position for three to five deep breaths. Return to a neutral position and repeat with the opposite leg. Extend your right leg up, keeping the knee bent. Ensure that your bent knee points downwards and the foot is flat against the side of the chair. Hold for three to five deep breaths, and then release. This pose is great for strengthening your lower body and can be done anytime, anywhere.

**Thigh/Hip Flexor**

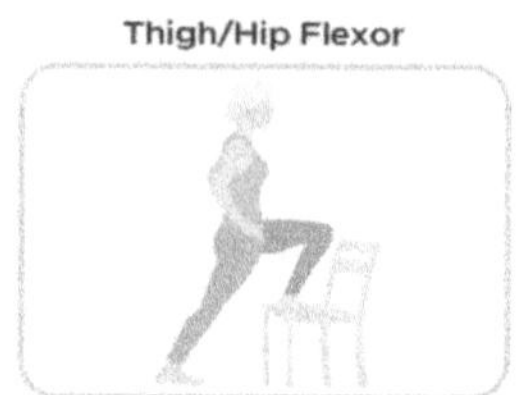

Hip Flexor Stretch - Improving Thighs, Hips, & Quadriceps: Begin by standing in front of a chair and place your hands on your hips. Lift your right foot and put it on the seat of the chair. Take a deep breath, and as you exhale, slowly lean forward, stretching your right quadriceps. Hold this position for two breaths and then return to your normal position. Switch sides and repeat the same steps with your left leg. Inhale slowly and place your left foot on the seat of the chair. Exhale as you slowly lean forward, stretching your left quadriceps. Hold for two breaths and return to normal.

Think again if you think flexibility can only be achieved through yoga on a mat. Chair yoga poses can make it abundantly clear that flexibility is not limited to traditional yoga practice. These poses are designed to make yoga accessible to everyone, regardless of physical limitations. As outlined here, a daily routine of gentle stretching and breathing can significantly improve your life. Aches, pains, and loss of flexibility don't have to be inevitable symptoms of aging that you have to endure. These issues can be addressed, improved upon, and sometimes even alleviated. And the best part is, you don't need complicated movements or intense exercises. A simple forward-bending chair yoga sequence can work wonders for flexibility. The body will become less stiff and more adaptable to movement when practiced regularly.

# Building Muscle Strength

"Old age isn't so bad when you consider the alternative." – Maurice Chevalier

Chair yoga is an effective way to improve flexibility and build muscle strength. While we have already talked about how chair yoga can improve flexibility, it is also essential to recognize the significance of building strength. As we age, our muscles gradually lose mass and effectiveness in supporting joints and bones. Therefore, it is not only about improving joint flexibility but also about fortifying the surrounding muscles. Muscle loss may start slowly and subtly, such as struggling while carrying groceries or getting tired after short walks. Once easy tasks become challenging, stamina may decrease faster. Other health conditions can also worsen muscle loss. Muscle weakening with age, called Sarcopenia, is primarily a natural process. However, exercise, especially resistance training, can help maintain and enhance strength, while diets rich in protein and essential vitamins benefit muscle health.

Maintaining muscle mass is essential for physical abilities and mobility, as muscle loss can negatively affect independence and freedom. However, a balanced diet and regular physical activity can help mitigate and even reverse some aspects of muscle loss. Consistent protein intake can also prevent further muscle loss. It is essential to take the proper measures. Although muscle loss is a natural part of aging, it can be controlled effectively. While diet does play a role in managing sarcopenia, physical exercise, especially resistance training, is the most effective countermeasure. Chair yoga, with its various poses, provides gentle resistance training. Although not the same as lifting heavy weights, it provides enough resistance to build and maintain strength by holding poses and using the body's resistance to shape and tone the muscles.

This chapter will explore these exercises in greater detail, offering you a balanced and less strenuous approach to physical activity. These strategic moves can help slow the effects of sarcopenia, making daily tasks easier and improving your overall quality of life. Let's get started!

To achieve maximum benefits, perform a sequence of gentle yet effective poses in a specific order. If any pose feels uncomfortable, listen to your body and focus on diaphragmatic breathing.

**Seated Twist:** Begin by sitting up straight in your chair. Exhale and place your right hand on your left knee while placing your left hand either behind your back or on the backrest of the chair. Gently twist your upper body to the left by using your hands. Hold this position for three breaths before returning to the centre. Repeat the same process on the other side by placing your left hand on your right knee and your right hand behind your back or on the backrest of the chair. Gently twist your upper body to the right by using your hands. Hold this position for three breaths and then return to the centre.

**Side Bend/Triangle**

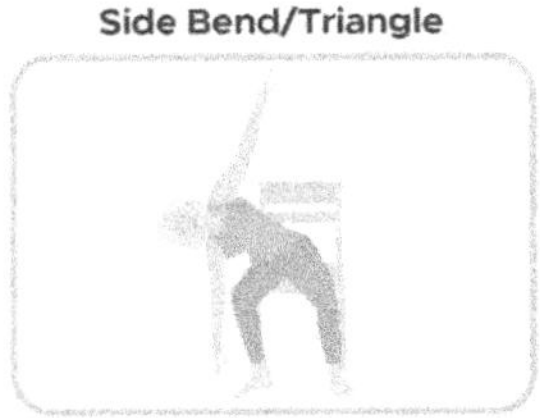

**Side Bend:** (Posture Enhancement) Side bend is a stretching exercise that requires you to maintain proper posture. Ensure that your shoulders, upper back, chest, and neck are aligned. Sit upright with your feet flat on the ground and extend both arms straight to your sides. Rotate your upper body to the left so that your left arm reaches towards the ceiling and your right arm extends towards the floor, which elongates the left side of your body. Hold this position for three breaths, then return to the center and repeat on the opposite side. Rotate your upper body to the right so that your right arm reaches towards the ceiling and your left arm extends towards the floor, stretching your right side. Hold for three breaths before returning to the center position.

**Leg Forward**

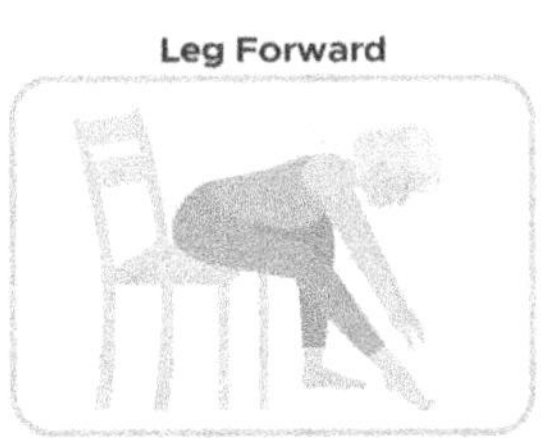

**Seated Forward Bend:** this is a yoga pose that can help enhance your strength and balance. To perform this pose, sit on the edge of your chair with both feet flat on the ground. Next, extend your right leg straight out with your heel resting on the ground and your toes pointing upward. Inhale and elongate your spine, then exhale and hinge at the hips to lean gently forward. You should feel a stretch along the back of your right leg. Hold this pose for three breaths, then switch to the other leg. Return to a neutral position, then extend your left leg straight out with your heel resting on the ground and toes pointing upward. Inhale and lengthen the spine, then exhale and hinge at the hips to lean forward gently. Feel the stretch along the back of your left leg.

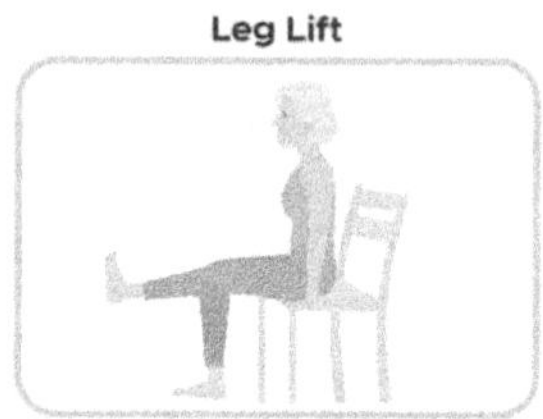

Leg Lift

**Leg Lifts:** Sit firmly in the chair with both feet flat. Lift each leg as straight as possible, hold for a count of ten, and then lower it. Repeat this three times for each leg. For added resistance, wear heavy shoes or boots.

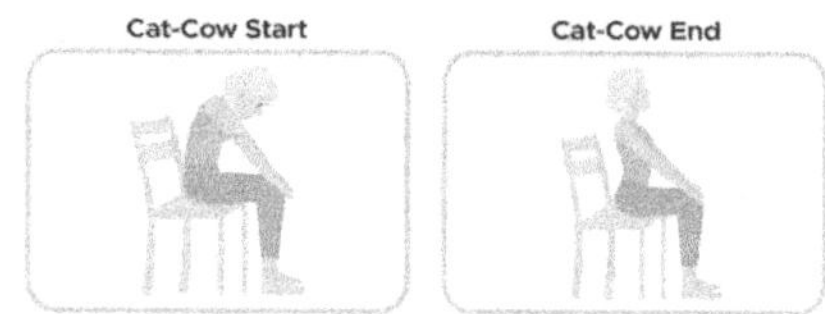

Cat-Cow Start     Cat-Cow End

**Cow-Camel Pose:** this is a great exercise for spinal flexibility. To do this, sit tall in your chair and place your hands on your thighs. As you exhale, round your back and tuck your chin towards your chest (Cow). Hold the pose for a few breaths, then slowly inhale and arch your back, lifting your chin and chest upwards (Camel). Alternate between these two poses for several breaths.

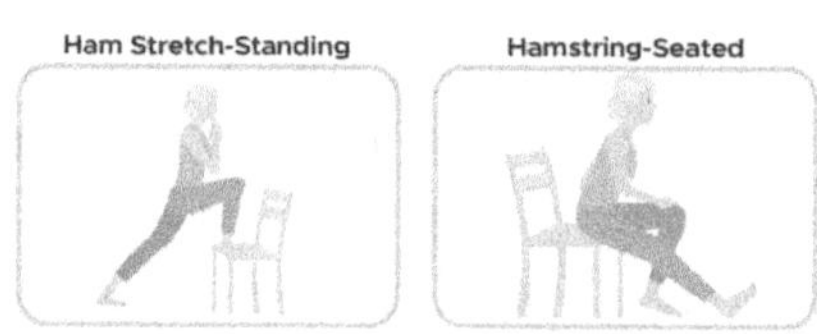

Ham Stretch-Standing     Hamstring-Seated

**Hamstring Stretch:** (Back and Hamstring) To perform a hamstring stretch, sit with both feet flat on the floor and legs at a 90-degree angle. Take your left leg forward and bend the left foot while maintaining the leg straight but not locked at the knee. Hinge at the hips while keeping your back straight and lean forward until you feel a stretch in the hamstrings. Hold this position for three breaths before switching sides. Now, extend your right leg forward and bend the right foot, maintaining the leg straight but not locked at the knee. Hinge at the hips while keeping your back straight and lean forward until you feel a stretch in the hamstrings. Hold this position for three breaths and return to the center. You can also perform this stretch while standing using a chair as support. In this case, make sure the leg being stretched is on the ground.

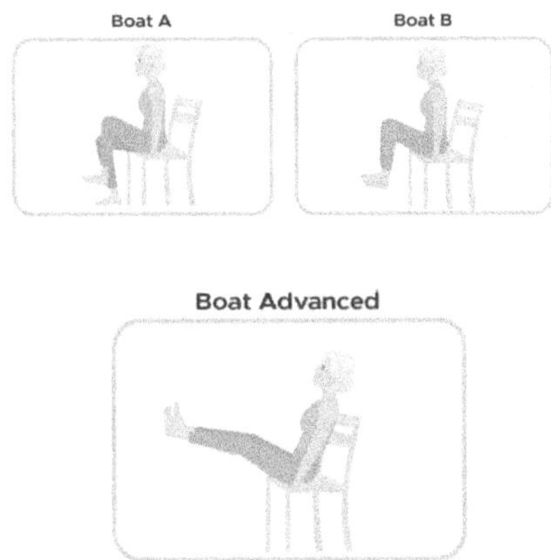


**Seated Boat Pose:** Begin by sitting in the middle of your chair with your feet flat on the floor, and use the sides of the chair for support. Lean back slightly and lift your left foot off the floor, followed by the right, bringing your knees towards your chest. Hold this position for several breaths before lowering your feet back to the ground. Repeat this movement four times, alternating the first leg lifted each time. For an added challenge, after several sessions, or for a more challenging workout, try extending both legs and lifting them until your body forms a "V" shape.

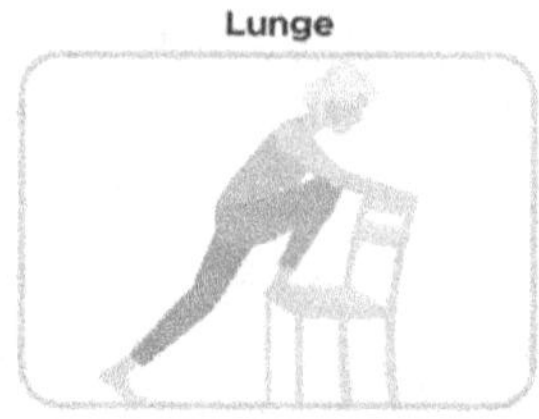



**Chair Stretches:** (Soothe Muscles, Relieve Leg, Groin, and Pelvic Pain)Chair stretches are a great way to stretch your legs while standing. Start by standing in front of a chair with your feet flat. Hold onto the back of the chair with both hands and place your left foot on the seat. Slowly push forward with your right leg and lean forward to stretch your left leg. Ensure your left knee aligns with your left ankle and let your hips sink slightly. Hold this position for three breaths before switching to your right leg.

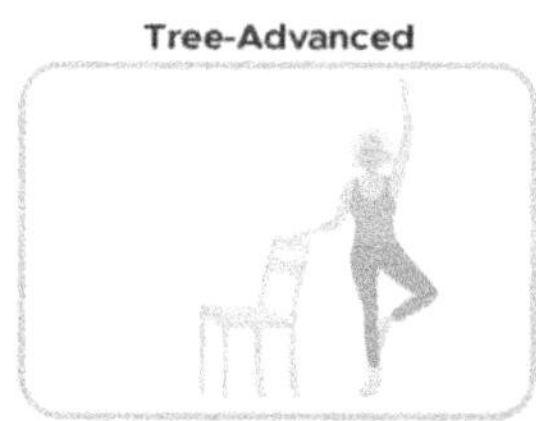



**Tree Pose:** Stand next to a chair and hold onto the backrest with your right hand for support. Place your right foot on the ground and lift your left foot. Put your left foot against your right leg's inner thigh or calf, but be careful not to touch your knee. Raise your left arm above your head and hold for a few breaths. Then, switch sides and repeat the same steps with your right foot.

Chair yoga can improve overall well-being and empower physical freedom. Combined with a balanced diet, it offers a holistic approach to managing aging-related changes.

# Improve your Balance

"Eventually you will reach a point when you stop lying about your age and start bragging about it." – Will Rogers

Enhancing Balance and Coordination in Later Years

As we age, maintaining balance and coordination can be a challenge. Falls can pose physical risks and jeopardize our independence. To prevent falls and maintain autonomy, we'll introduce you to chair yoga exercises designed to enhance balance and coordination.

The Objective of Chair Yoga

Chair yoga promotes comfort and stability within your current capabilities, improving balance and coordination. It enhances physical health, autonomy, and the joy of living. Exercises that require muscle groups to work together improve physical strength and motor skills, aiding in regaining physical independence. Maintaining balance becomes challenging as we age, impacting daily functions. Chair yoga offers an effective means to enhance coordination and equilibrium without imposing excessive strain on the body.

Understanding Balance Mechanisms

Our brain, nerves, muscles, and sensory systems may not coordinate well as we age, resulting in balance issues. Medications for age-related conditions can further impact balance. Recognizing declining balance and taking prompt action to maintain well-being is crucial.

Beyond Aging: Understanding Balance Challenges

Many health conditions can disrupt balance besides natural aging. Inner ear problems, alcohol, diabetes, and peripheral neuropathy are among the factors contributing to balance issues. Poor balance affects the quality of life, curtails activities, and instills fear of falling. It's intricately linked to overall well-being, and circulatory and breathing problems can also affect balance.

Various factors, such as low blood sugar levels, inner ear problems, hearing loss, and impaired vision can cause vertigo. These can all impact balance and make tasks like walking more difficult.

Maintaining balance can profoundly impact daily life, leading to a cautious approach to activities and potentially fostering a less active life-style. Physical inactivity, in turn, can contribute to various health issues, including cardiovascular diseases and depression.

How Chair Yoga Can Aid Balance

Consult your doctor first if you're experiencing balance issues. Chair yoga is a valuable tool for enhancing overall health and balance. It offers complementary benefits by improving muscle tone and strength, aiding in balance maintenance despite medical challenges. Necessary tests and medical history reviews can identify underlying conditions impacting balance, which can be addressed through medication, physical therapy, or lifestyle changes. Incorporating balance exercises into daily routines can also be highly beneficial when performed regularly.

The Potential of Chair Yoga

Chair yoga is a convenient way to improve balance and coordination, especially for those who find traditional yoga or exercise challenging. It combines strength training, flexibility, and breath regulation, offering a holistic approach to balance. Mindful breathing practices help calm the mind and enhance balance-related cognitive functions. Research shows chair yoga improves muscle tone, flexibility, and body awareness, leading to better proprioception. Balancing requires a harmonious interplay of various systems, and exercises like chair yoga serve as potent tools to improve balance.

## Exercises for Coordination and Balance

This routine aims to enhance coordination and balance by incorporating a variety of movements and breathing patterns that can be easily integrated into daily routines or performed as a full practice. If you find a pose too challenging or uncomfortable, Modify poses or try diaphragmatic breathing if needed. Focus on your breathing and take your time. Chair Yoga is an individual practice that emphasizes personal growth, stability, and inner calm. Start slowly and progress as you get more robust and more comfortable.

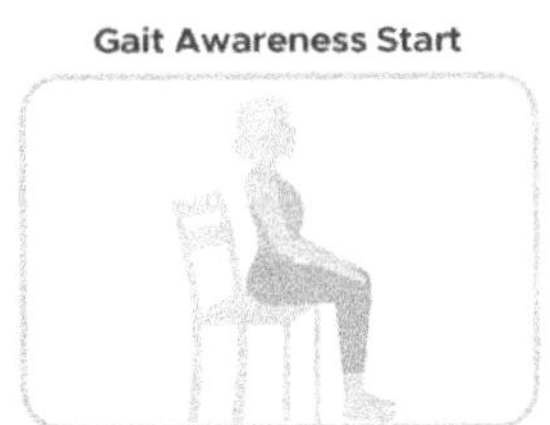


**Purification Breathing:** This is a technique that can help revitalize the body and restore balance. Start sitting comfortably with your back straight and feet flat on the floor to do this technique. You can close your eyes if you prefer. Place your hands on your knees and inhale deeply and slowly through your nose, allowing your chest and abdomen to expand. Next, exhale forcefully but in a controlled way through your mouth while drawing your abdomen in. Repeat this breathing pattern for a few cycles to experience its benefits.

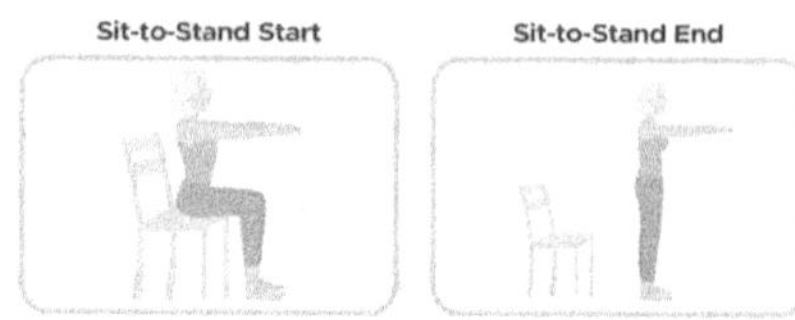


**Sit-to-Stand (Targets Thighs and Lower Body):** The Sit to Stand pose is great for strengthening your legs and improving your coordination during transitions. If performed vigorously, it can also serve as a cardiovascular exercise. To start, sit at the front edge of a sturdy chair and position your feet flat on the floor, approximately hip-width apart. You can place your hands on your thighs or the chair's armrests. Lean forward slightly and push into your hands while straightening your legs to stand up. Slowly reverse the movement and sit back down. Repeat this sequence of movements in rapid succession for a set of repetitions.

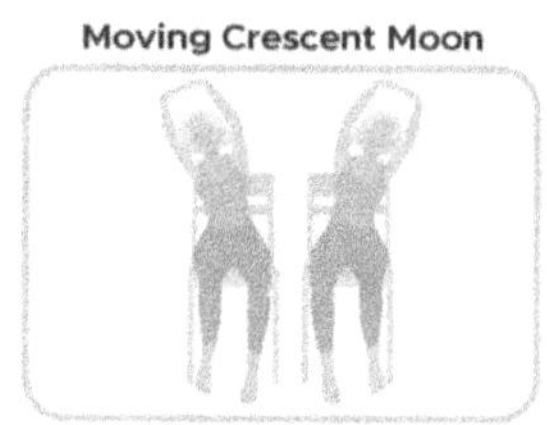


**Seated Crescent Moon Pose (Posture, Core, and Spine):** Seated Crescent Moon is a yoga pose that can be practiced while sitting on a chair. To perform this pose, sit upright and extend both arms overhead, clasping your hands together. Lean your body to the right and hold for two breaths. Inhale while returning to the center, exhale, lean your body to the left, and hold for two breaths. Inhale while returning to the center, exhale, and repeat the left-right stretch several times. This pose is excellent for stretching the sides of your body and can be done anytime to relieve tension and improve posture.

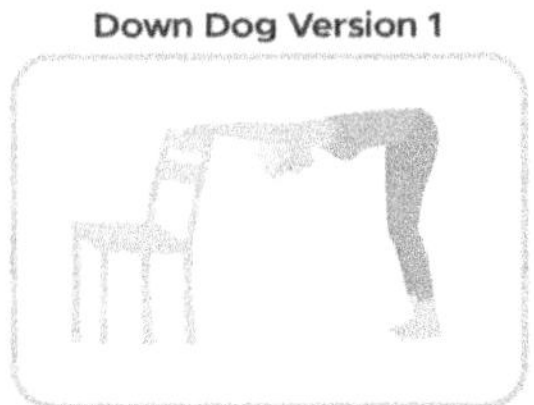

Down Dog Version 1

**Chair Downward-Facing Dog Pose (Targets Shoulders, Core, and Spine):** Stand facing the back of a sturdy chair, keeping approximately an arm's length away. Spread your fingers wide and place them on the back of the chair. Step your feet back until your arms are stretched straight, forming an inverted V shape with the body. Press your hips back and down, keeping your feet flat on the floor. Hold this position for ten breaths. Alternatively, you can perform this pose facing the front with your hands on the seat.

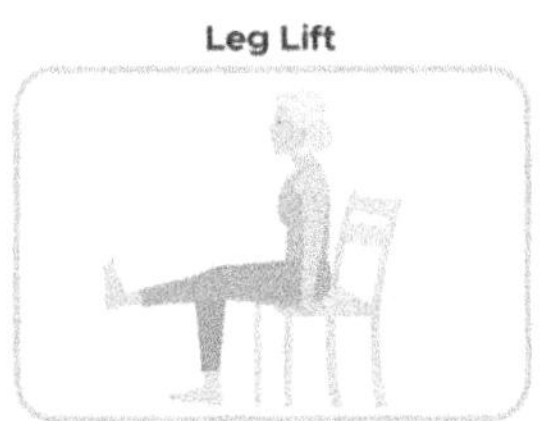

Leg Lift

**Leg Lifts (Targets Abs, Quads, and Core):** Leg lifts are a great way to strengthen your quadriceps and improve your balance. Start by sitting upright in a chair with both feet firmly planted on the floor to do this pose. Straighten your right leg and lift it to hip height while keeping your knee straight. Hold your leg in the raised position for three breaths, then lower it back to the floor. Repeat the same steps with your left leg.

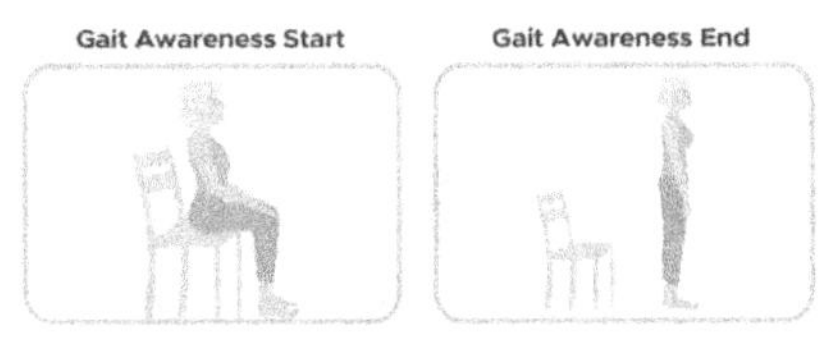

Gait Awareness Start    Gait Awareness End

. . .

**Awareness Pose (Balancing):** The Awareness pose is designed to improve your balance, coordination, and stability. It involves a slow and purposeful balancing act. To begin, sit on a chair with your hands resting on your thighs. Then, stand up with your back facing the chair. Carefully lift your right knee towards your chest, and step forward with your right foot, placing your heel down first. Shift your weight onto your right foot and lift your left foot, stepping it forward similarly. Repeat this walking movement for several steps, then turn around and do it again in the opposite direction.

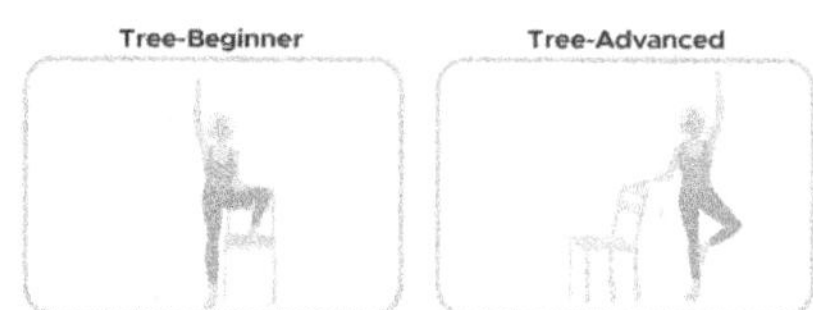


**Tree Pose (Focus: Balance)** The Tree pose is an excellent yoga pose that helps target different body parts, such as your legs, core, hips, inner thigh, and groin. To perform this pose, you must stand beside a chair and hold onto the backrest with your right hand for support. Next, place your right foot flat on the ground and lift your left knee onto the chair beside you. Optionally, you can put the sole of the lifted foot against the inner thigh or calf of the standing leg, avoiding the knee area. Then, bring your left arm above your head and hold for several breaths. Finally, repeat the same steps for the opposite side.

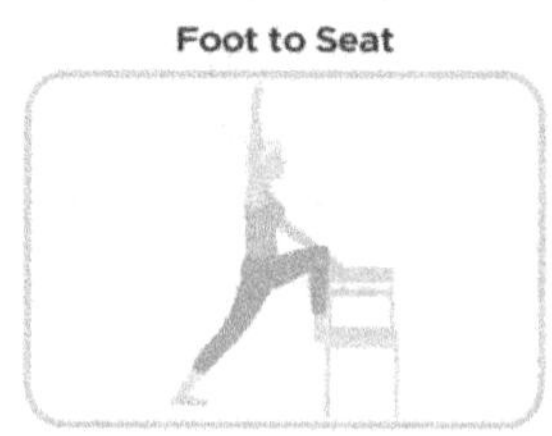


**Foot-to-Seat Pose (Targets Legs, Hips, Shoulders, and Back):** Assuming the "Foot to seat pose" position involves standing beside a chair, approximately two steps away from it. Next, place your right hand on the back of the chair and step your left foot onto the seat. Then, extend your left arm overhead, pointing your fingers. Hold this position for three breaths, and you should feel a good stretch along the side of your body. This pose is excellent for opening up the side body and improving balance. To repeat on the other side, grasp the chair with your left hand, step your right foot onto the seat, and extend your right arm overhead.

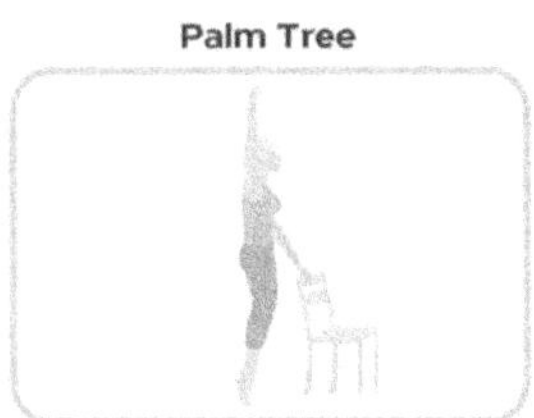

**Palm Tree**

**Palm Tree Pose (Focus: Palms, Legs, Knees, Back, and Neck)**Stand facing the back of a chair and hold onto the backrest with your left hand. Rise onto the balls of your feet and stretch your right arm overhead, feeling the stretch on the side of your body. Then, return your hand to the chair and flatten your feet. Repeat the same steps on the opposite side: hold onto the backrest with your right hand, rise onto the balls of your feet, and stretch your left arm overhead, feeling the stretch on the side of your body. Hold this position for a few seconds before returning to the starting position. This pose is excellent for improving balance, strengthening the calf muscles, and stretching the side body.

# Pain Management

"You know you're getting old when the candles cost more than the cake." – Bob Hope

Chronic pain can arise from various sources, such as musculoskeletal disorders, neurodegenerative disorders, peripheral disorders, and other conditions. Arthritis is an example of a musculoskeletal disorder that can cause significant discomfort. Neurodegenerative disorders, such as Parkinson's disease and multiple sclerosis, affect the brain and nerves over time, while peripheral disorders affect the extremities like hands and feet. Changes in the brain's pain processing mechanism can also occur as one ages, leading to a heightened perception of pain. Chronic pain can also be a secondary symptom of chronic conditions like diabetes, heart disease, and kidney failure.

Chronic pain can impact a person's life, leading to reduced physical activity, poor sleep, and affect mental health. It's essential to get a thorough assessment from healthcare professionals and tailor a treatment plan to individual needs. Exercise and lifestyle changes often are the backbone of at-home pain management strategies. Yoga is increasingly recommended for pain relief as it focuses not just on the site of the pain but aims to bring balance to the entire body, reducing pain and minimizing the risk of injuries. Stretching exercises are also recommended as an alternative to more strenuous exercises and prescription medications, improving flexibility and aiding in the range of motion, often compromised in chronic pain conditions.

Here are some commonly recommended chair yoga exercises that can help relieve pain:

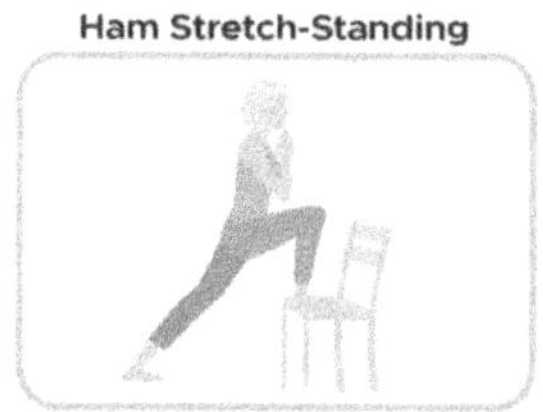


**Hamstring Stretch:** This stretch can ease lower back and leg pain. Sit at the edge of a chair and extend one leg in front of you with your heel on the floor.

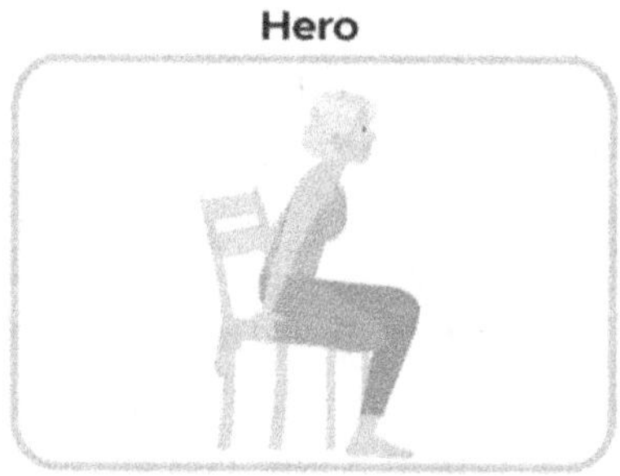


**Quadriceps Stretch:** This stretch is helpful if you experience knee pain. Stand next to a wall and hold onto a chair for support. Gently pull one foot towards your buttocks. If you prefer a seated version, try the "Hero's Stretch."

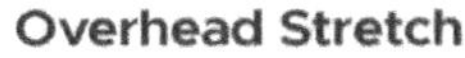



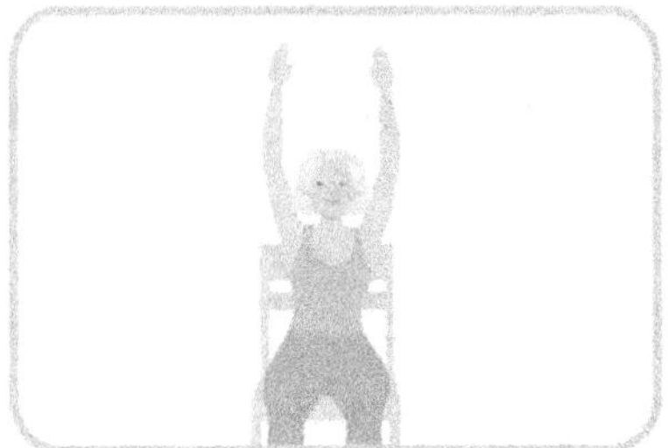

**Arm and Shoulder Stretch:** This stretch is helpful if you experience discomfort in your upper body. Stretch out your arms and rotate your wrists and shoulders.

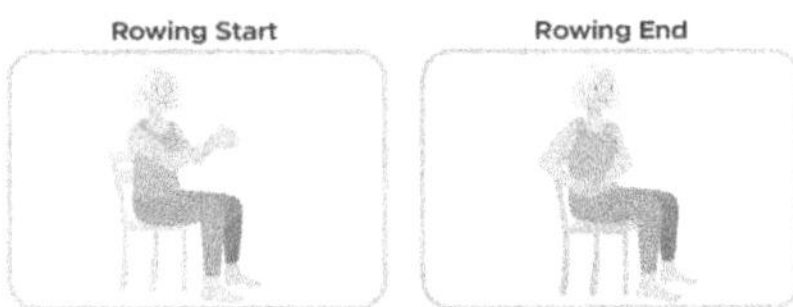



**Spinal Twist:** This stretch is good for back pain. Gently rotate your spine from side to side. If you prefer a gentle version, try the Rowing Movement.

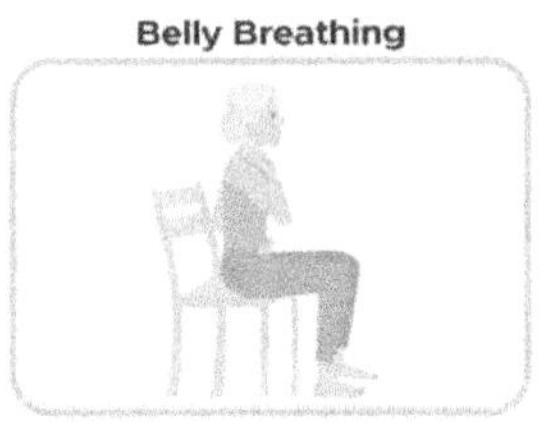



**Deep Breathing and Relaxation:** While not technically a stretch, deep, mindful breathing can relax tense muscles often associated with chronic pain.

Methods that encompass both stretching and holistic approaches, such as yoga, play a significant role in managing neuropathic or nerve-related pain. However, it is essential to remember that any self-administered treatment at home should be integrated into a comprehensive pain management plan, typically devised after a thorough evaluation by healthcare professionals. Tailoring the treatment to suit individual needs is crucial for optimal effectiveness, as each individual's condition is unique.

Managing neuropathic pain can be complex because the intricate network of nerves transmits various signals, including pain, between the body and the brain. Neuropathic pain can stem from a range of conditions, such as spinal cord injuries, diabetes, and other nerve-related ailments.

Yoga can help manage neuropathic pain through multiple avenues. First, it aids in calming the nervous system, thereby alleviating the heightened sensitivity often associated with neuropathic pain. Second, yoga promotes the release of endorphins, the body's natural pain relievers. Finally, the practice emphasizes controlled breathing, which has its own set of benefits. Deep, measured breaths can induce a relaxation response, helping alleviate stress and reduce nerve sensitivity.

Role of Nutrition

Yoga can help manage chronic pain, while nutrition can also play a key role. Certain foods can either worsen or alleviate pain. Before starting yoga or any exercise, consult your healthcare provider, especially if you have specific medical conditions. Please pay attention to your body and avoid pushing it beyond discomfort. Take breaks and practice diaphragmatic breathing if needed.

**Pain Relief Exercises**

Specially designed poses in this sequence target areas particularly beneficial for alleviating pain:

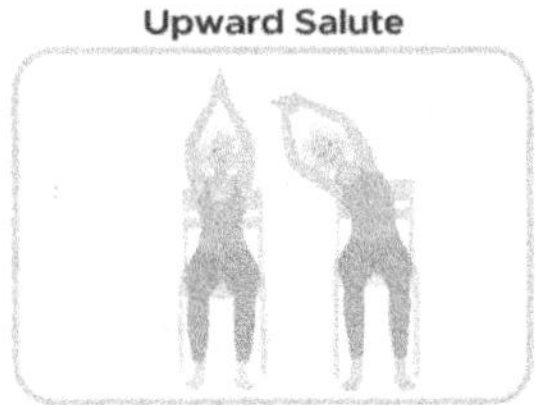

Upward Salute

**Upward Salute for Hips, Back, and Shoulders:** "Upward Salute" is an outstanding yoga pose. To do this pose, sit straight with your feet flat on the floor. Inhale and raise your arms overhead, keeping your palms facing each other. You can look straight ahead or upward, but be careful not to strain your neck. Hold this position for three to five breaths, then slowly lower your arms as you exhale.

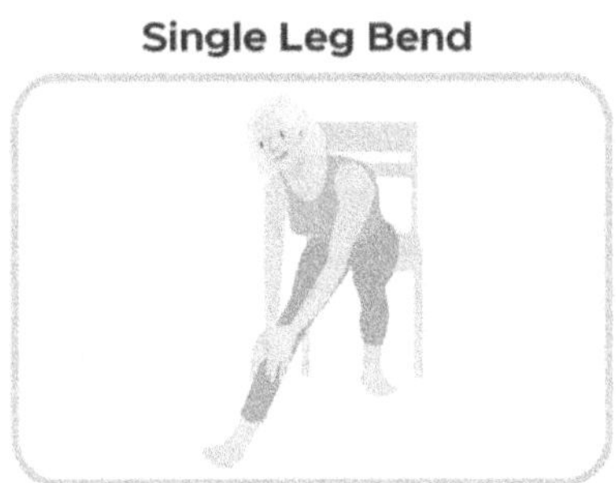

Single Leg Bend

**Single Leg Stretch for Hamstrings, Glutes, and Back:** Sit close to the edge of your chair and extend your right leg straight. Inhale to prepare. As you exhale, hinge at the hips and lean forward to stretch the hamstring of the extended leg. Hold for three to five breaths, then switch sides.

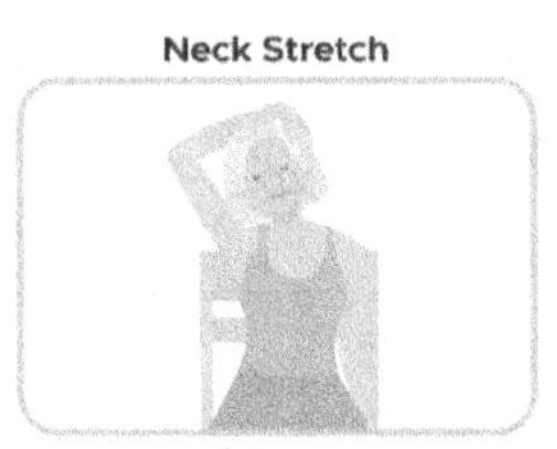

Neck Stretch

**Neck Tilts:** To perform the neck tilts exercise, keep your back straight and place your left hand on the right side of your head. Inhale through your nose and gently tilt your head towards your left shoulder. Hold the pose for two breaths as you exhale through your mouth and then return to the center. Repeat this two times. Switch to the right side, placing your right hand on the left side of your head. Inhale through your nose and gently tilt your head towards your right shoulder. Exhale and hold the pose for two breaths. Repeat the exercise for each side.

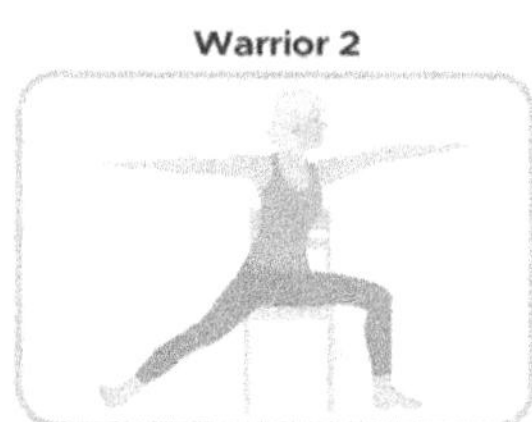


**Warrior 2:** Assume Warrior 2 pose by turning your torso to face the front of the chair while extending your arms to the sides like an airplane, palms facing down. Take three deep breaths, inhaling and exhaling—transition to Reverse Warrior.

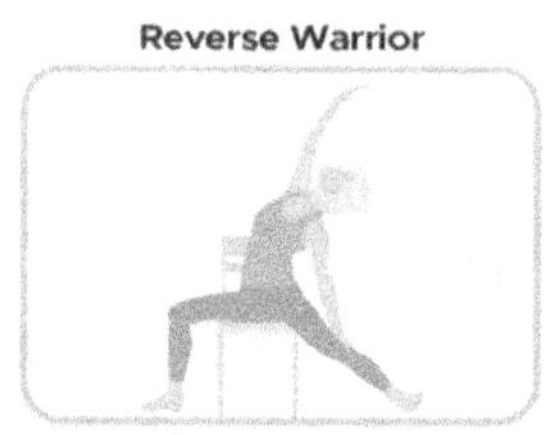


**Reverse Warrior:** Reverse Warrior is a yoga pose where you lower your left hand down towards your left foot while lifting your right hand and bending it slightly over your head. This helps to open up the chest and side of the body. It would be best if you held this pose while focusing on four deep breaths. If the Warrior poses are too strenuous, it is recommended that you pause for a brief rest or practice diaphragmatic breathing before moving on to the next exercise.

Inversions, where the head is below the heart, can be challenging and unsuitable for everyone. If you find inversions uncomfortable if they are contraindicated for your health condition, or if you find it difficult to transition from one pose to the next, take a break and practice diaphragmatic breathing. This technique involves deep breathing that engages the diaphragm, encouraging full oxygen exchange. It's an excellent way to relax the nervous system and can be used as a break between any two poses in the sequence.

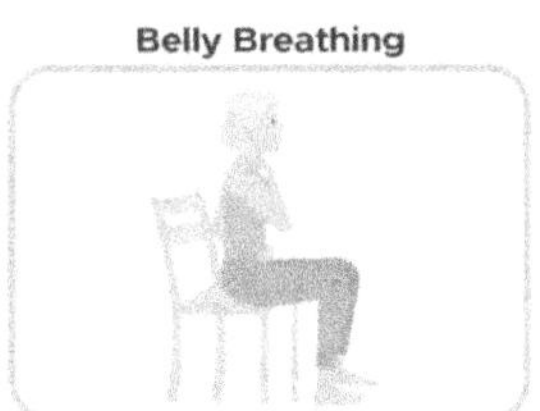


**Diaphragmatic breathing** is a relaxation technique that involves breathing deeply and slowly to help calm your mind and body. To perform this exercise, get comfortable and place one hand on your chest and the other on your abdomen. Inhale deeply through your nose, allowing your abdomen to rise as you fill your lungs with air. Then, exhale slowly and fully through your mouth, noticing the descent of your abdomen. Repeat this cycle a few times until you feel relaxed and prepared to proceed.

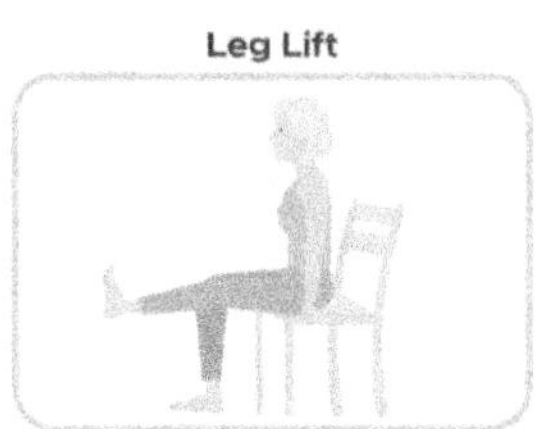


**Leg Lifts:** A helpful exercise for people experiencing knee pain during squats is sitting firmly in a chair with both feet flat on the ground. Engage your core and raise one leg to keep it as straight as possible. Hold this position for a count of three, then lower your leg back down.

Repeat the exercise by alternating legs, aiming for 4-9 repetitions on each side.

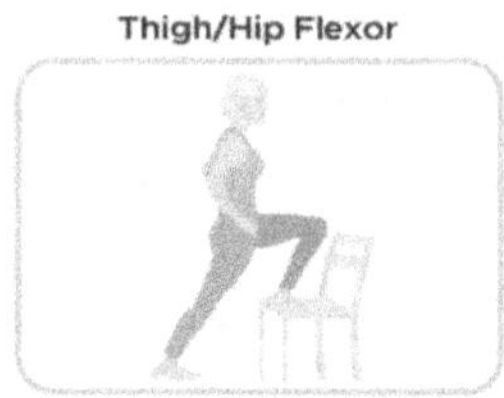


**Hip Flexor stretch:** This is a helpful exercise for those who spend long periods sitting down and suffer from hip pain. Start by standing in front of a chair. If you have balance issues, hold onto a second chair for support. Keep your left foot firmly on the ground and extend your right leg, placing your right foot onto the chair seat. Keep your spine straight as you gently push your hips forward, feeling a stretch along the front of the extended leg. Take deep breaths and hold this position for several breaths before switching sides. Carefully place your right foot on the ground and position your left leg on the chair seat. Keep your spine straight as you gently push your hips forward, feeling a stretch along the front of the extended leg. Repeat this exercise 7-10 times, alternating between sides.

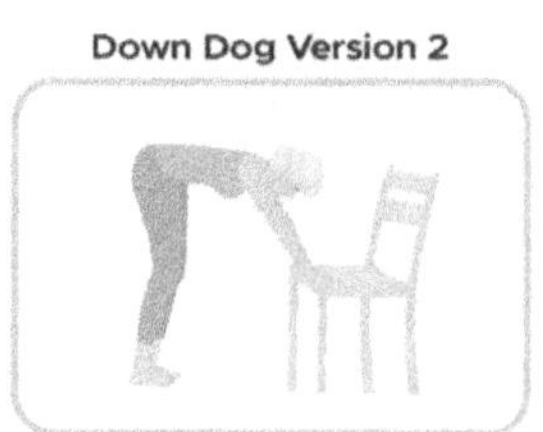


**Downward dog with Chair:** Downward dog with Chair Stretch for Back, Hamstrings, and Shoulders: Place your hands on the chair seat or on the top edge of the backrest. Push the chair back as you lean forward, extending your arms and lowering your head between them. Ensure your back forms a straight line from your tailbone to your head. Hold the position for three to four breaths, feeling the stretch along your spine, shoulders, and hamstrings.

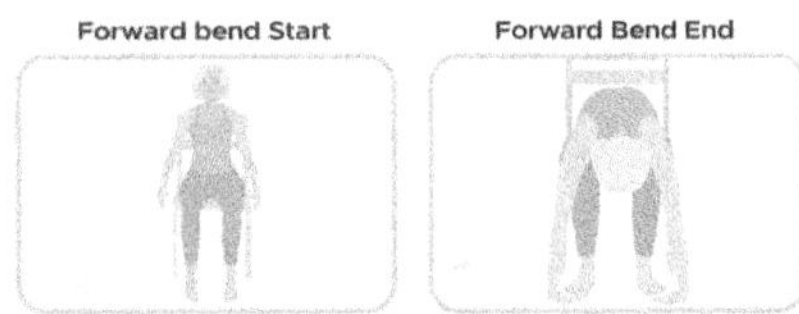



**Forward Bend:** The Forward Bend yoga pose primarily targets the sciatic nerve, calf muscles, hamstrings, and inner thigh adductors. To perform this pose, you must stand upright on a sturdy chair with your feet flat. As you take a deep breath, hinge at the hips and fold forward while exhaling. You can reach for the floor with your palms up or let your hands rest on your knees. Stay in a comfortable forward bend for 30 seconds to a minute while breathing slowly. Finally, slowly roll back up to the seated position.

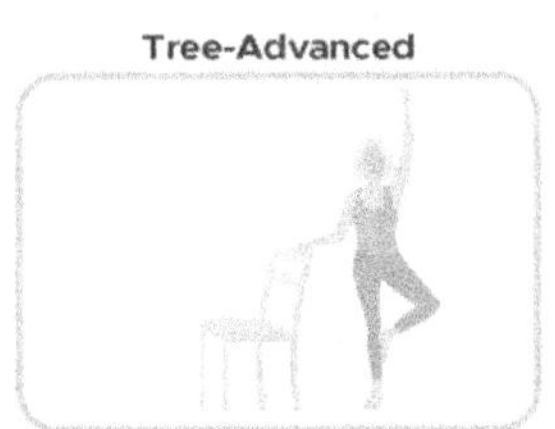



**Tree Pose:** Tree Pose for Hip and Inner Thigh Pain: Stand next to the back of the chair with your right hand on the chair's back. Lift your left foot and place the sole on the inner right thigh or calf, avoiding putting it on the knee joint. Raise the left arm into a crescent moon shape. Breathe deeply and hold for several breaths, then switch sides. Place your left hand on the chair's back, lift your right foot, and place the sole on the inner left thigh or calf, ensuring you avoid putting it on the knee joint. Raise the right arm into a crescent moon shape. Breathe deeply and hold for several breaths. Repeat both sides two times.

**Seated Eagle**

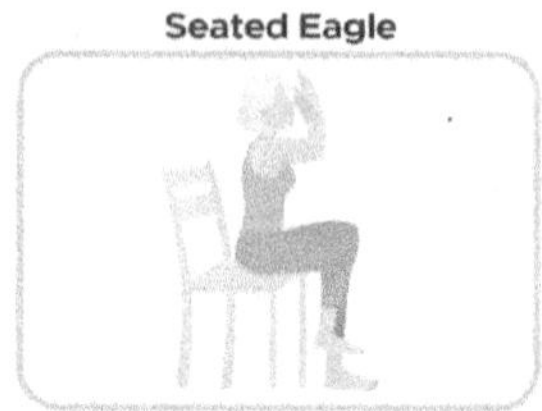

**Seated Eagle:** Seated Eagle for Back Pain: This yoga pose focuses on the back, hips, and shoulders. To do this pose, sit upright with your feet flat on the floor. Bring your hands together and keep your elbows close. Twist your right arm around your left, touching your palm to your left. Keep your spine straight and shoulders relaxed. Cross your right leg over your left. Look straight ahead or close your eyes. Inhale deeply through your nose, hold for three seconds, and exhale through your mouth. Repeat for three breaths, relaxing on the final exhale.

To switch sides, bring your hands together and elbows close. Twist your left arm around your right, palms touching. Keep your back straight and shoulders relaxed. Cross your left leg over your right. Look straight ahead, inhale deeply through your nose, holding for three seconds. Exhale through your mouth and repeat three times, relaxing on the final exhale.

Alternate Version: Arms only, without crossing your legs.

**Pigeon**

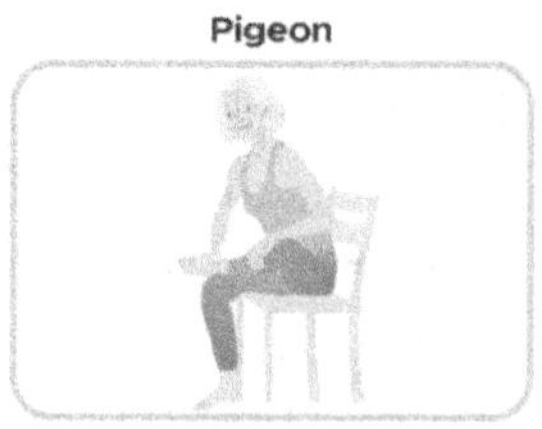

**Pigeon Pose:** Pigeon Pose is a great way to improve mobility, lower back pain, and hip flexibility. To start, stand upright with both feet flat on the floor. Lift your left ankle over your right thigh, creating a figure-four shape. Make sure to point your left knee outwards as much as possible. If you feel comfortable, gently press down on the left knee for a deeper stretch. Hinge at the hips and lean forward slightly to increase the stretch further, keeping your back straight. Hold this pose for several breaths, then switch to the other side. Lift your right ankle and place it over your left thigh, pointing your right knee outwards as much as possible. If comfortable, gently press down on the right knee for a deeper stretch. Hold this pose for several breaths and then relax.

**Seated Triangle**

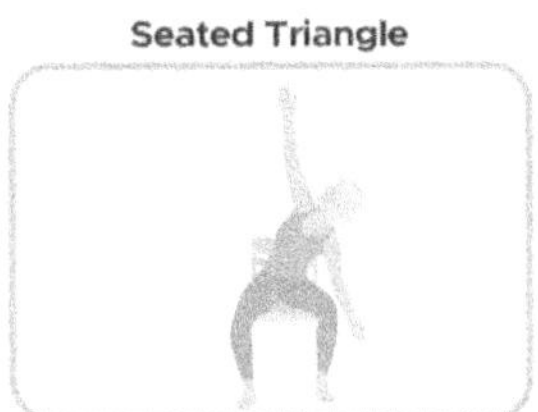

**Triangle:** To perform the Triangle exercise for your torso obliques and intercostal muscles, sit upright at the edge of your chair with your legs shoulder-width apart. Extend your arms to the sides, palms facing downwards like an airplane. Then, bend at the waist and lean to your right, reaching your right hand towards your right ankle while your left arm points upwards. You can look up or straight ahead, whichever is comfortable for your neck. Take deep breaths and hold the position for several breaths before switching to the other side.

On the other side, extend your arms to the sides, palms facing downwards like an airplane. Incline at the waist and lean to the left this time, reaching your left hand towards your left ankle while your right arm points upwards. Try to gaze upwards or look straight ahead if that strains the neck. Take deep breaths and hold for several breaths. Repeat on both sides.

Our 28-day workout plan is designed to improve your physical and emotional health. This partnership can improve your life by offering increased mobility, strength, and flexibility - attributes that are physical and psychological cornerstones of a joyful life. The plan aims to provide a stronger, more flexible, and cheerful self and is an open invitation to everyone who seeks to cultivate a life where joy holds the reins.

# 28 Days to double Fitness

"The older I get, the better I used to be." – Lee Trevino

Welcome to a transformative journey towards doubling your fitness and vitality through the power of chair yoga. In this chapter, we'll embark on a 28-day exploration of chair yoga, designed specifically for individuals over 60 but ultimately beneficial for people of any age. Through gentle yet effective yoga poses, breath work, and mindfulness practices, you'll discover how to enhance your physical fitness, flexibility, and overall well-being from the comfort of your chair.

## Day 1: Setting Intentions

As we begin our 28-day chair yoga journey, it's essential to set clear intentions for what we hope to achieve. Take a moment to reflect on your goals and aspirations for the next four weeks. Whether you aim to improve flexibility, build strength, reduce stress, or incorporate more movement into your daily routine, clarifying your intentions will help guide your practice and keep you motivated throughout the journey.

## Day 2-7: Foundations of Chair Yoga

During the first week of our chair yoga program, we'll focus on laying the foundations for a strong and sustainable practice, try to remember the movements without relying on the diagram, towards the end of the routine we will remove some diagrams because you will have done them so often they will be set in your mind. Each day, we'll explore fundamental yoga poses, breathing techniques, and mindfulness practices that form the building blocks of chair yoga. From seated stretches to gentle twists and mindful breathing exercises, you'll learn how to connect with your body, breath, and mind in new and transformative ways.

## Day 8-14: Strength and Stability

In the second week of our chair yoga journey, strength and stability in both body and mind will improve. Through dynamic seated poses and resistance exercises, you'll engage your muscles, improve balance, and enhance core strength.

## Day 15-21: Flexibility and Flow

As we enter the third week of our chair yoga program, you will improve in flexibility and fluidity of movement. Through various seated stretches, gentle twists, and flowing sequences, you'll gradually release tension, improve your range of motion, and cultivate a sense of ease and openness in your body.

## Day 22-28: Integration and Transformation

In the final week of our chair yoga journey, we'll integrate all that we've learned and experienced over the past three weeks. You'll deepen your connection to yourself and the present moment through a series of holistic practices that combine movement, breath, and mindfulness. As you continue to nurture your body, mind, and spirit, you'll witness the transformative power of chair yoga unfold, leading to greater fitness, vitality, and overall well-being.

## Conclusion: Celebrating Your Progress

As our 28-day chair yoga program comes to a close, take a moment to celebrate your progress and accomplishments. Whether you've noticed improvements in flexibility, strength, balance, or feel more centered and grounded, every step forward is a testament to your dedication and commitment to your health and well-being.

You will be ready to test yourself again

Here are some important points to consider:

Rest Days: Rest days are strategically incorporated throughout the plan, Breathing exercises are on these days to maintain mindfulness and relaxation.

If you miss more than two consecutive days, it is recommended that you restart the plan from Day 1 to get back on track and maximize your benefits.

The program lasts for 28 days, but you should continue your exercise routine even after completing it. You can repeat the plan or concentrate on your preferred sections. Furthermore, you can use certain exercises to tackle any new problems that arise. So, let's begin this journey together.

**28-Day Chair Yoga Routine**

READ THROUGH THE MOVEMENTS BEFORE YOU START

This section offers a comprehensive 28-day chair yoga routine to boost your confidence and skills, suitable for beginners and those with experience. The step-by-step guide prioritizes simplicity and ease of use. Practicing a few minutes daily for 28 days makes yoga less intimidating and more enjoyable. This routine enhances physical strength, flexibility, and mental relaxation, promoting overall well-being. The sequences are designed to last 5-15 minutes, easily fitting into a busy schedule or combining for longer sessions. Use the downloadable chart of poses provided. Let's start!

**Day 1:** Warm-Ups: Perform as many repetitions as you feel comfortable with.

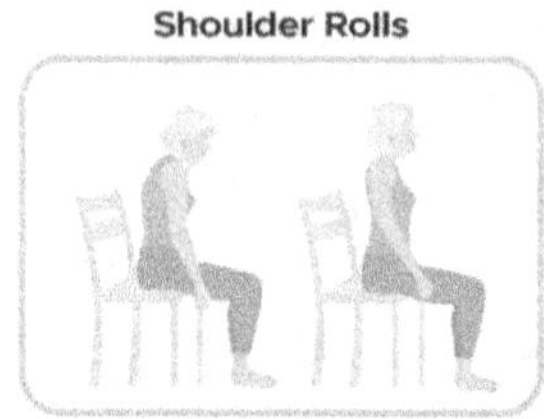



**Shoulder Rolls:** To do shoulder rolls, close your eyes and slowly lift your shoulders up towards your ears while inhaling. Then, roll them back and down while exhaling. Repeat this movement in a clockwise and counterclockwise direction, while being mindful of your breath. This exercise can help to release tension in your shoulders and improve your posture.

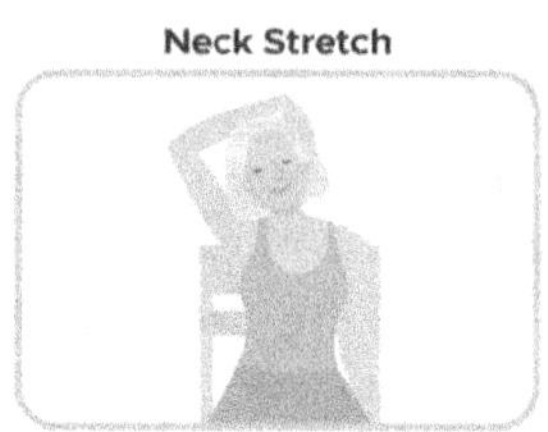



**Neck Tilts:** While keeping your back straight, gently tilt your head towards your left shoulder. Hold for two breaths, then return to the center. Repeat on the right side. Perform this twice on each side.

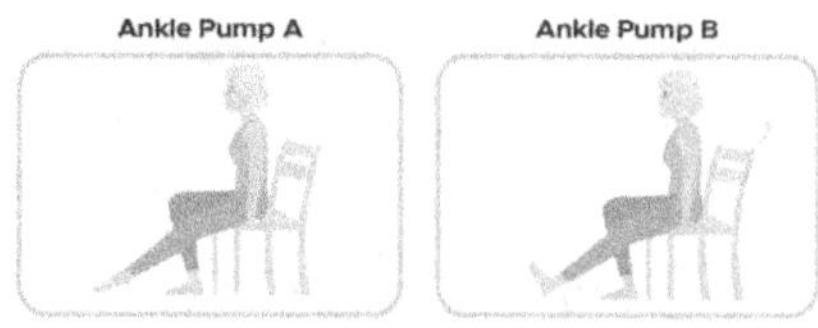



**Ankle Pumps:** Perform ankle pumps by lifting heels and toes alternately, repeating five times. Remember to breathe.

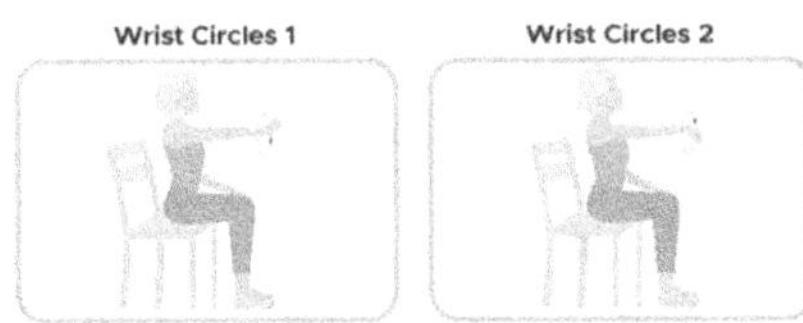

**Wrist Circles:** Extend your arms in front with palms facing down. Begin rotating your wrists clockwise for five rotations, then counterclockwise for another five.

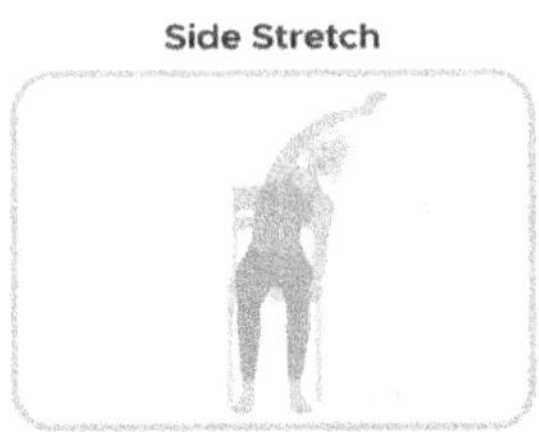

**Side Stretch:** Extend your arms overhead while inhaling. While exhaling, lean to the left side for a gentle stretch. Return to the center while inhaling, then lean to the right while exhaling. Repeat this twice on each side.

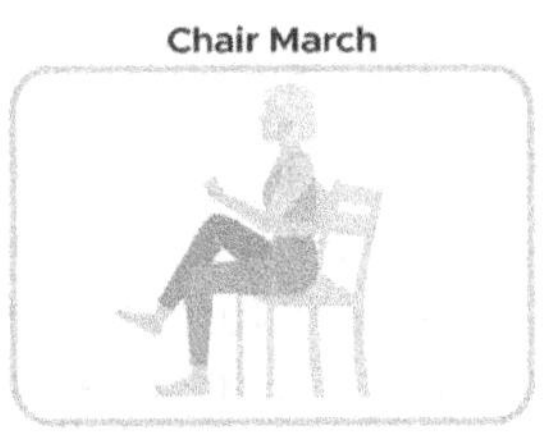

**Chair March:** This can also be done standing next to your chair. Sit up straight with your feet on the floor and arms bent at the elbows. Begin by lifting your right foot and left arm up while pushing your right arm back. Transition to left arm and right foot up as if you were marching. Continue this motion for 3 minutes at a moderate pace.

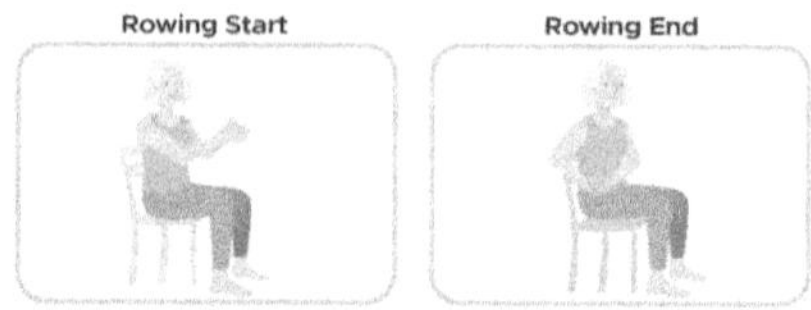


**Seated Rowing:** Start by sitting forward in your chair. Clasp your hands together and stretch them out in front of you to your left side. "Paddle" your hands from front to back at a medium speed as if you are rowing a canoe. Repeat this movement five times, then switch to the right side and repeat. Perform the entire sequence four times.

**Day 1 - Main Sequence:**

**Belly Breathing (Control your Breathing)**

Settle into a comfortable seat position with a straight back. Place one hand on your chest and the other on your belly. Inhale deeply through your nose, letting your belly expand while keeping your chest still. Hold for a moment, then exhale slowly through your mouth, feeling your belly draw inward. Repeat for ten breaths, focusing on your belly's rhythmic rise and fall. Experience the calming effect as you fully engage in this mindful breathing exercise.

**Ocean Sounding Breath (Concentration)**

Sit upright with relaxed shoulders and gently inhale through your nose. As you exhale, slightly constrict the back of your throat to produce a soft, soothing sound reminiscent of ocean waves or fogging a mirror. Aim to create this tranquil sound during both inhalation and exhalation. Repeat this calming practice 5-10 times, letting the gentle oceanic rhythm guide your breath and enhance your focus.

By beginning with these foundational exercises, you're setting the stage for a rewarding and transformative journey through chair yoga. Consistency is key, and with time and dedication, you'll see remarkable progress. So, let's embark on this journey together, unlocking the myriad benefits of chair yoga and enhancing your well-being along the way.

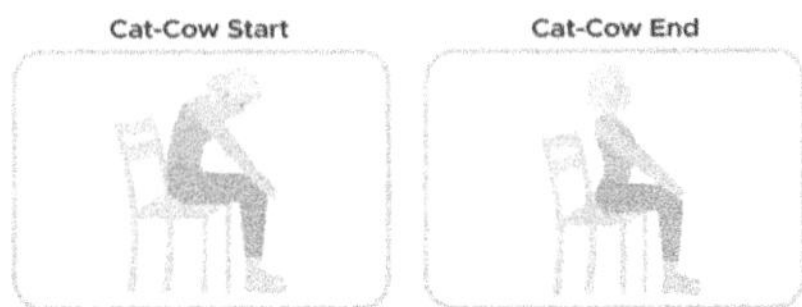



**Cat-Cow Pose:** Return to a seated position with your back straight and both feet planted firmly on the floor. Place your hands on your knees, grounding yourself in the present moment. Inhale deeply as you arch your back and look up, stretching the front of your neck. Exhale slowly as you round your back, tucking in your chin and stretching the back of your neck. Flow through this sequence for ten cycles, synchronizing your movements with your breath to enhance balance, posture, and flexibility.

## Upward Salute

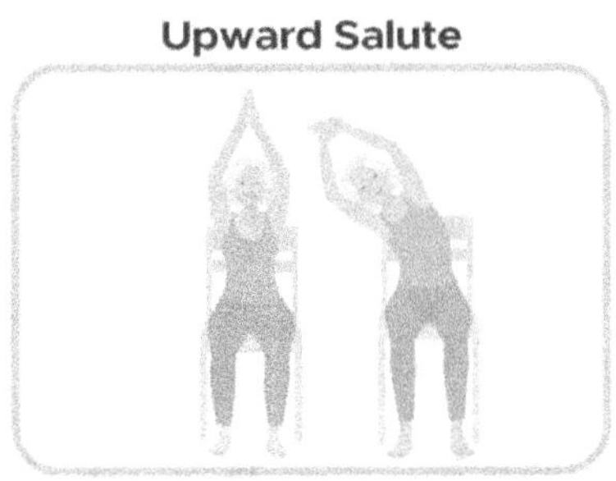

**Salute to the Sun:** Sit upright with your feet flat on the floor, grounding yourself in the present moment. Inhale deeply as you extend your arms overhead, palms facing each other. Gaze straight ahead or upwards without straining your neck. Hold this pose for three to five breaths, feeling the energy coursing through your body before gracefully lowering your arms on the exhale.

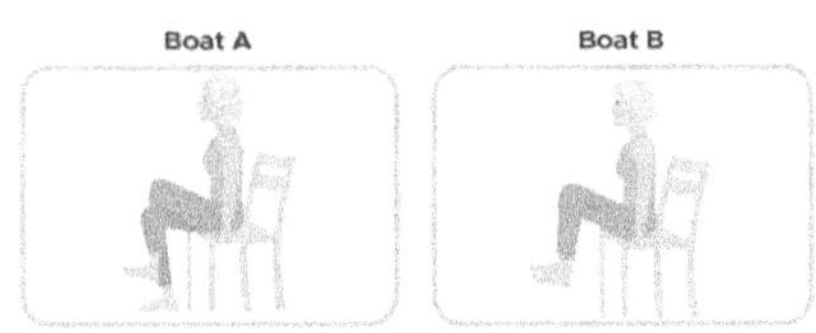

. . .

**Seated Boat Pose:** Shift your focus inward as you transition to Seated Boat Pose. Find the middle of your chair and plant your feet firmly on the floor for stability. Hold onto the sides of the chair for support as you lean back slightly. Lift your left foot off the floor, followed by the right, drawing your knees towards your chest. Feel the engagement in your core and the deep stretch in your hip flexors. Hold this pose for several breaths before gently lowering your feet back to the ground. Repeat this sequence four times, alternating the first leg on the ground each time to achieve balance and symmetry.

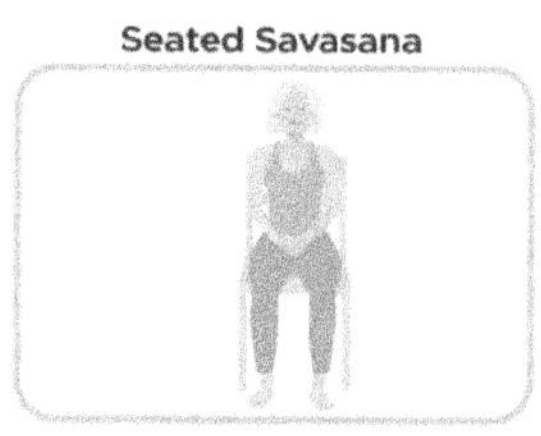

Seated Savasana

**Chair Savasana:** Transition into a state of deep relaxation with Chair Savasana. Sit comfortably with your back straight, feet flat on the ground, and hands resting in your lap. Close your eyes and allow your body to relax completely, starting from your head and neck, down through your arms and torso, all the way to your legs and feet. Breathe naturally, letting go of tension with each exhale. Remain in this serene posture for about three minutes, allowing yourself to experience a profound sense of calm and inner peace.

**Day 2:** Warm-Ups: Begin your practice with gentle warm-up exercises to prepare your body and mind for the day ahead.

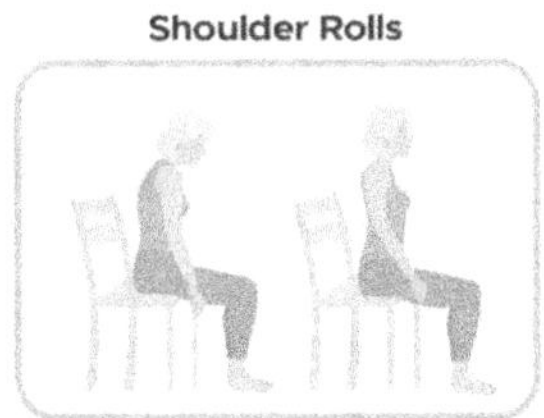


**Shoulder Rolls:** To do shoulder rolls, close your eyes and slowly lift your shoulders up towards your ears while inhaling. Then, roll them back and down while exhaling. Repeat this movement in a clockwise and counterclockwise direction, while being mindful of your breath. This exercise can help to release tension in your shoulders and improve your posture.

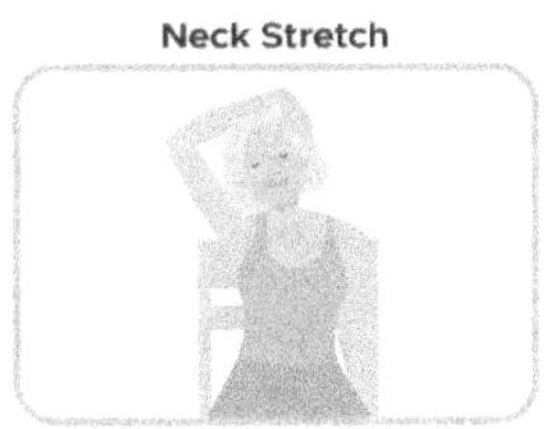


**Neck Tilts:** While keeping your back straight, gently tilt your head towards your left shoulder. Hold for two breaths, then return to the center. Repeat on the right side. Perform this twice on each side.

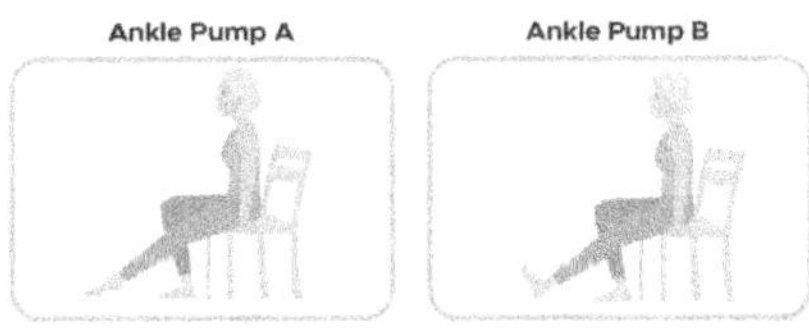


**Ankle Pumps:** Perform ankle pumps by lifting heels and toes alternately, repeating five times. Remember to breathe.

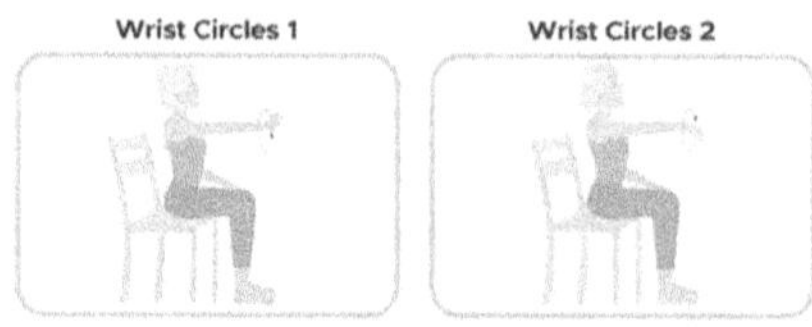

**Wrist Circles:** Extend your arms in front with palms facing down. Begin rotating your wrists clockwise for five rotations, then counter-clockwise for another five.

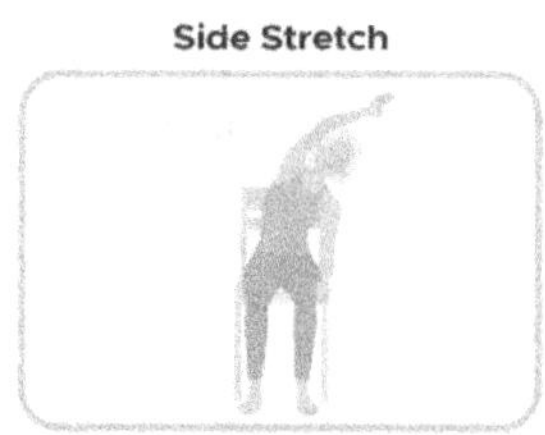

**Side Stretch:** Extend your arms overhead while inhaling. While exhaling, lean to the left side for a gentle stretch. Return to the center while inhaling, then lean to the right while exhaling. Repeat this twice on each side.

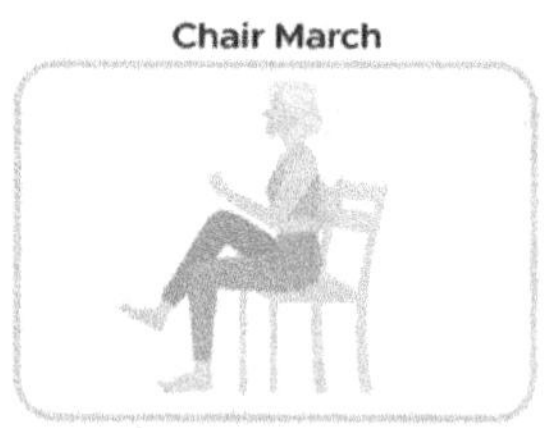

**Chair March:** This can also be done standing next to your chair. Sit up straight with your feet on the floor and arms bent at the elbows. Begin by lifting your right foot and left arm up while pushing your right arm back. Transition to left arm and right foot up as if you were marching. Continue this motion for 3 minutes at a moderate pace.

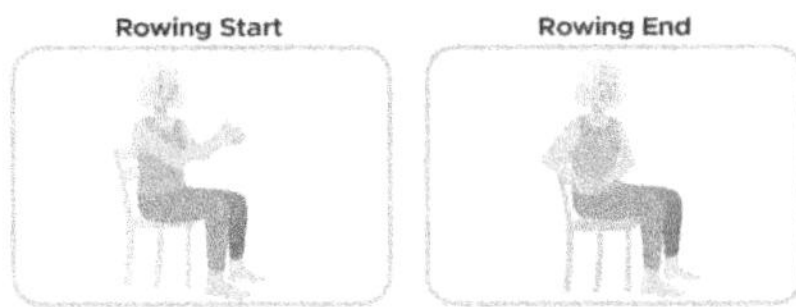



**Seated Rowing:** Start by sitting forward in your chair. Clasp your hands together and stretch them out in front of you to your left side. "Paddle" your hands from front to back at a medium speed as if you are rowing a canoe. Repeat this movement five times, then switch to the right side and repeat. Perform the entire sequence four times.

By dedicating time to your chair yoga practice each day, you're investing in your physical and mental well-being, cultivating resilience, strength, and inner peace. Remember to listen to your body and honor its needs as you embark on this transformative journey. With each breath and movement, may you find greater ease, balance, and joy in your life.

**Day 2 - Main Sequence:**

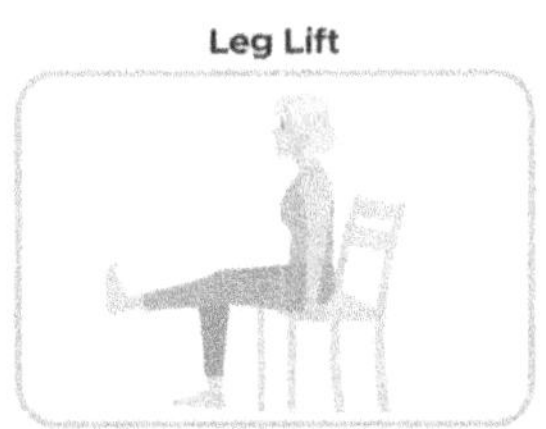



**Leg Lifts (Quadriceps, Abs):** firmly in your chair with both feet flat on the ground, gripping the sides for stability. Inhale slowly, lifting your left leg and keeping it as straight as possible. Hold for a count of five, feeling the engagement in your quadriceps and abs. Exhale as you lower your leg. Repeat three times, then switch to your right leg. Inhale slowly, lifting your right leg straight. Hold for a count of five, then exhale as you lower it. Repeat five times for each leg. For added resistance and a greater challenge, wear heavy shoes or boots. Feel the strength and power building with each lift.

**Ham Stretch-Standing**

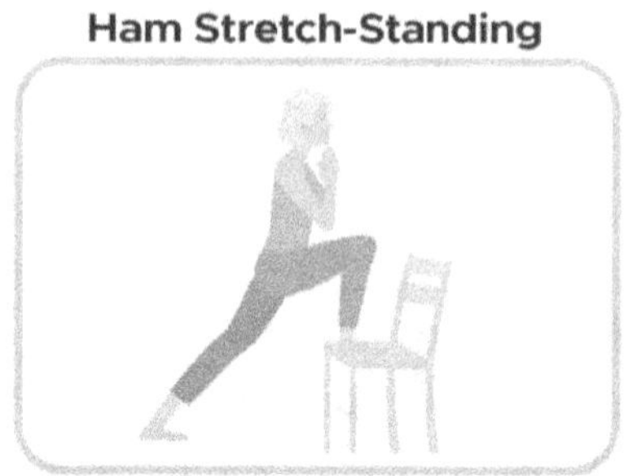

**Hamstring Stretch (Lower Back, Hamstrings):** Stand gracefully in front of the chair. Extend your right leg forward, placing it gently on the seat while keeping your left leg grounded on the floor. With elegance, bend forward and hinge at the hips, maintaining your spine's graceful alignment until you sense a gentle stretch in your left hamstring. For added poise and support, lightly grasp the chair back. Embrace this moment of stretch and relaxation for three soothing breaths before gracefully transitioning to the other side.

**Side Bend/Triangle**

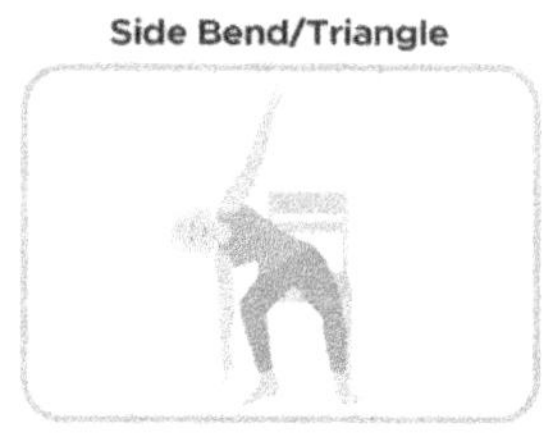

**Side Bend (Posture, shoulders, upper back, chest, neck):** Sit straight with your feet flat on the ground, ensuring your spine is tall and aligned. Extend both arms straight out to your sides, parallel to the floor, with your palms facing down. Inhale deeply, and as you exhale, bend to your left, reaching your left arm toward the ceiling and your right arm toward the floor. Feel the stretch along the entire left side of your body, from your fingertips down to your hip. Hold this pose for three deep breaths, allowing your body to relax into the stretch.

After three breaths, gently return to the center, bringing both arms back to shoulder height. Take a moment to realign and inhale deeply once more. On your next exhale, bend to your right, this time reaching your right arm toward the ceiling and your left arm toward the floor. Stretch the right side of your body, feeling the elongation and release of tension. Hold this position for three deep breaths, focusing on the stretch and maintaining steady, even breathing.

Finally, return to the center position, bringing your arms back to shoulder height. Take a moment to relax and feel the balance and alignment in your body. Repeat this sequence as needed to promote flexibility and relieve tension along the sides of your body.

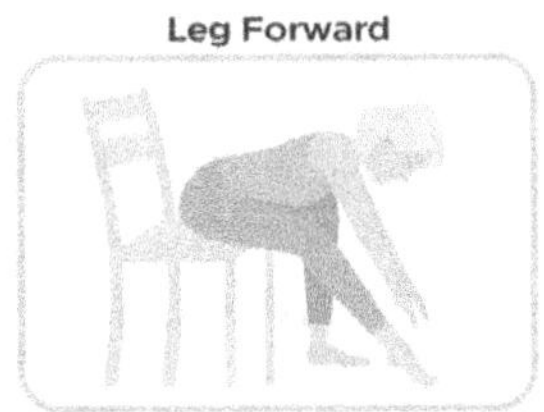

Leg Forward

**Leg Forward Bend (Core Strength, Balance, Lower Back, Hamstrings):** Sit on the edge of your chair with your feet flat on the ground, poised and ready. Extend your right leg straight out, resting your heel on the ground and pointing your toes up. Inhale deeply, feeling your spine lengthen and your posture lift. As you exhale, hinge forward at the hips, leaning into the stretch and feeling the tension release from your hamstring. Hold this invigorating stretch for three deep breaths. Return to a neutral position, savoring the alignment, then repeat the sequence with your left leg, enjoying the stretch and the sense of balance it brings.

**Raised Hands**

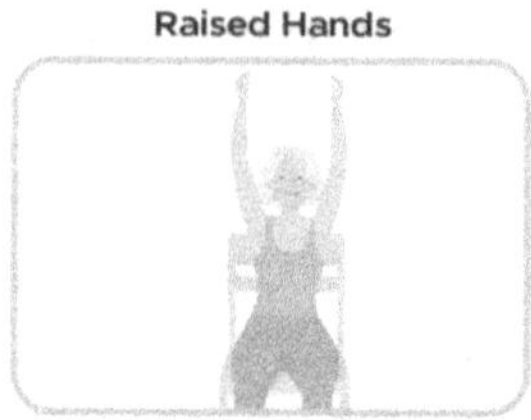

**Raised Hands Pose (Arms, Shoulders, Upper Back, Chest):**Sit comfortably with your back straight and feet flat on the floor, feeling grounded and poised. Inhale slowly, raising your arms above your head, aligning them with your ears as much as possible. Keep your shoulders relaxed and avoid hunching. Feel the stretch and openness in your upper body. Hold this empowering pose for three to five deep breaths, savoring the stretch and the calm it brings. As you exhale, slowly lower your hands back to your lap, feeling a sense of relaxation and balance.

## Day 3: Rest Day/ Mindful Breathing

**Relaxing Breathing Techniques for Focus and Peace**

**Box Breathing:** Inhale gently through your nose, counting to four. Hold your breath for four counts. Exhale slowly through your mouth for four counts. Hold the exhale for another count of four. Repeat this rhythmic cycle 5-10 times to promote calmness and center your mind.

**Ocean Breath:** Find a comfortable seated position with relaxed posture. Inhale deeply through your nose, maintaining closed lips. Exhale through your nose while gently constricting the back of your throat, creating a soft, soothing sound reminiscent of ocean waves. Practice this tranquil technique 5-10 times to enhance focus and mindfulness.

**Belly Breathing:** Sit comfortably with a straight back. Place one hand on your chest and the other on your belly. Inhale deeply through your nose, allowing your belly to expand while keeping your chest still.

Exhale slowly through your mouth, drawing your belly inward. Continue for a few minutes, focusing on the gentle rise and fall of your belly to promote relaxation and ease stress.

**Ocean Sounding Breath:** Sit upright with relaxed shoulders. Inhale slowly through your nose, then exhale through your nose while gently constricting the back of your throat. Aim for a soft, whisper-like sound during both inhalation and exhalation, similar to fogging a mirror. Repeat this calming exercise ten times to cultivate a sense of peace and clarity.

**Humming Breath (Calming, Stress Relief):** Close your eyes and take a slow, deep breath through your nose. Exhale slowly through your mouth while humming softly. Repeat this soothing practice 5-10 times to calm your mind and release tension.

**Day 4 - Warm ups:** Warm-Ups: Perform as many repetitions as you feel comfortable with.

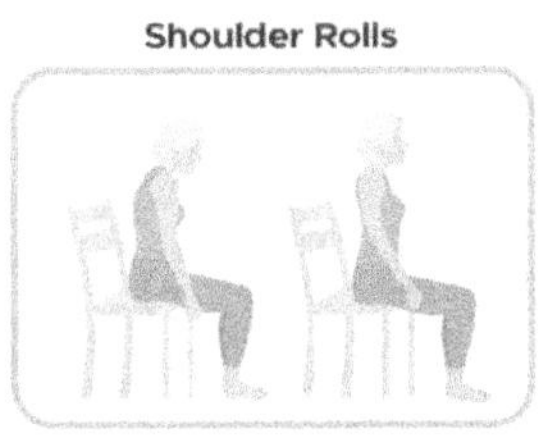


**Shoulder Rolls:** To do shoulder rolls, close your eyes and slowly lift your shoulders up towards your ears while inhaling. Then, roll them back and down while exhaling. Repeat this movement in a clockwise and counterclockwise direction, while being mindful of your breath. This exercise can help to release tension in your shoulders and improve your posture.

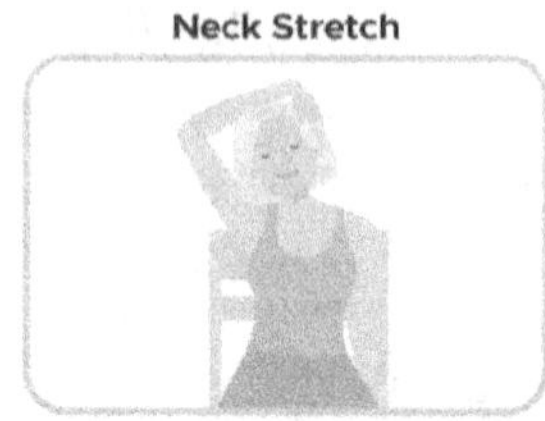

Neck Stretch

**Neck Tilts:** While keeping your back straight, gently tilt your head towards your left shoulder. Hold for two breaths, then return to the center. Repeat on the right side. Perform this twice on each side.

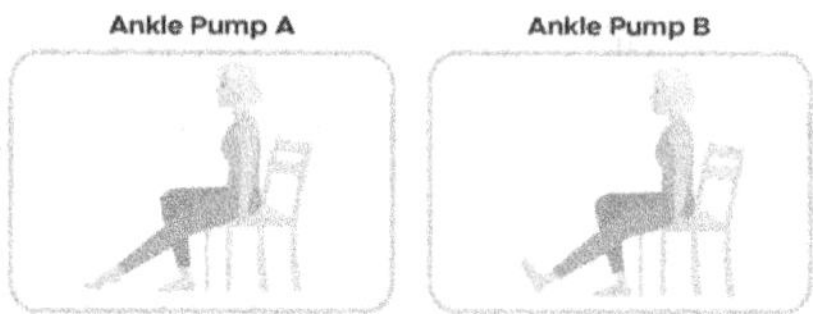

Ankle Pump A      Ankle Pump B

**Ankle Pumps:** Perform ankle pumps by lifting heels and toes alternately, repeating five times. Remember to breathe.

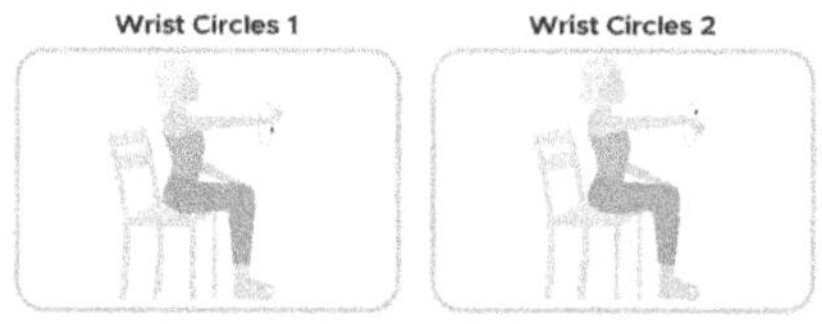

Wrist Circles 1      Wrist Circles 2

**Wrist Circles:** Extend your arms in front with palms facing down. Begin rotating your wrists clockwise for five rotations, then counterclockwise for another five.

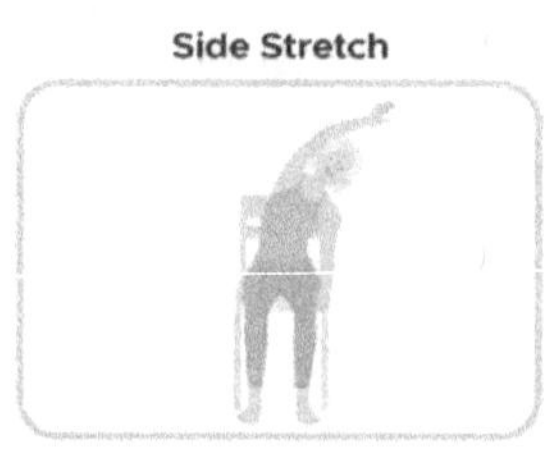

Side Stretch

**Side Stretch:** Extend your arms overhead while inhaling. While exhaling, lean to the left side for a gentle stretch. Return to the center while inhaling, then lean to the right while exhaling. Repeat this twice on each side.

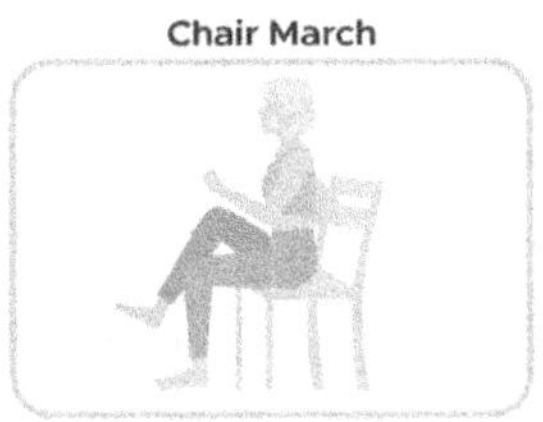

Chair March

**Chair March:** This can also be done standing next to your chair. Sit up straight with your feet on the floor and arms bent at the elbows. Begin by lifting your right foot and left arm up while pushing your right arm back. Transition to left arm and right foot up as if you were marching. Continue this motion for 3 minutes at a moderate pace.

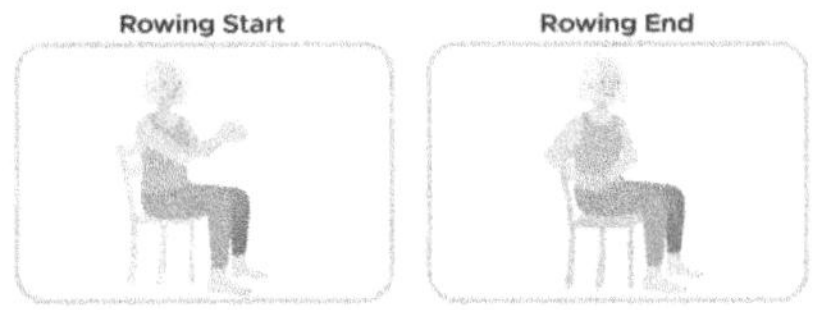

Rowing Start          Rowing End

**Seated Rowing:** Start by sitting forward in your chair. Clasp your hands together and stretch them out in front of you to your left side. "Paddle" your hands from front to back at a medium speed as if you are rowing a canoe. Repeat this movement five times, then switch to the right side and repeat. Perform the entire sequence four times.

**Day 4 - Main Sequence:**

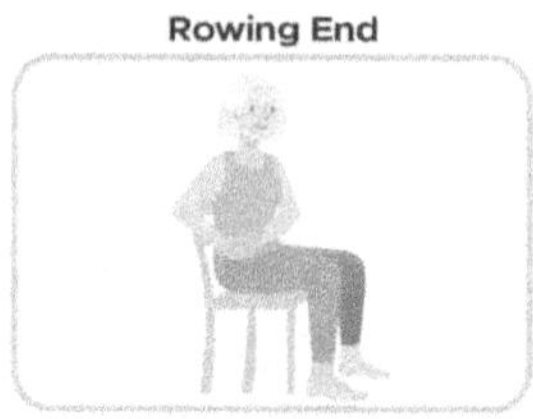



**Seated Twist (Spine):** Start by sitting with your back straight. As you exhale, place your left hand on your right knee and your right hand behind you, either on the backrest or the chair. Use your hands to twist your upper body to the right gently. Hold the twist for three deep breaths, feeling the stretch along your spine. Return to the center and repeat on the other side for balance and flexibility.

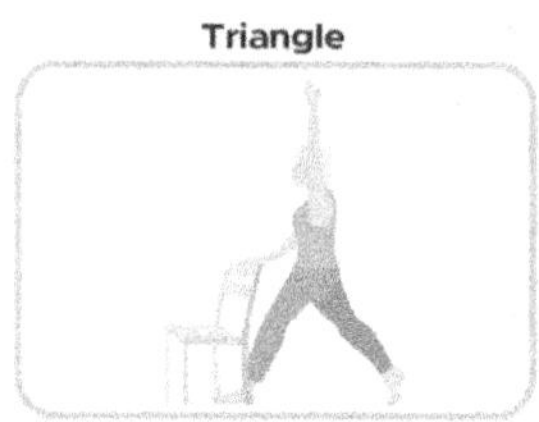



**Triangle Pose (Torso, Spine, Abdominals, Intercoastal Muscles):** Begin by standing beside your chair with the backrest to your right. Place your feet slightly under the chair and spread them shoulder-width apart. Hold onto the chair back with your right hand as you step your right foot back about three feet. Extend your left arm up toward the ceiling, creating a long line from your fingertips to your back heel. Breathe deeply and hold the pose for several breaths, feeling a stretch through your torso and intercostal muscles. Transition to the other side and repeat for symmetry and alignment.

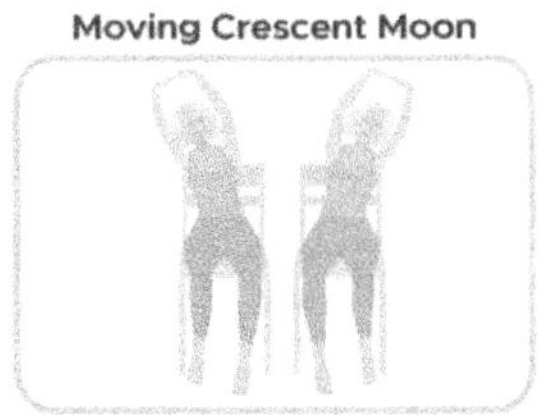

Moving Crescent Moon

**Crescent Moon Pose (Posture, Core, Spine):** Sit upright in your chair and stretch your left arm overhead in a gentle curve. Lean your body to the right, elongating through your left side. Hold this stretch for two deep breaths, feeling a soothing lengthening from your fingertips down to your hip. Inhale as you return to the center, then exhale and repeat on the other side. Stretch your right arm overhead and lean to the left, focusing on elongating your right side. Hold for two breaths, then inhale back to center. Repeat the left-right stretch sequence several times to enhance flexibility and ease tension.

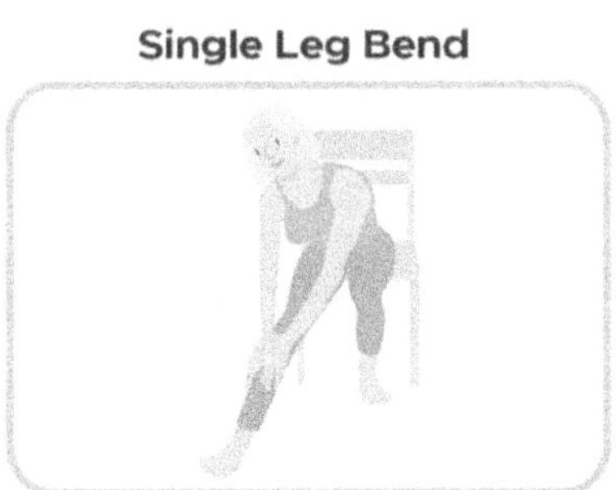

Single Leg Bend

**Single Leg Stretch (Hamstrings, Glutes, Back):** Sit close to the edge of your chair and extend your right leg straight out in front of you. Inhale to prepare, then exhale as you hinge at the hips and lean forward, stretching the hamstrings of your extended leg. Hold the stretch for three to five breaths, feeling the lengthening sensation in your leg muscles. Switch sides and repeat, ensuring both legs receive equal attention and flexibility benefits.

Single Leg Balance

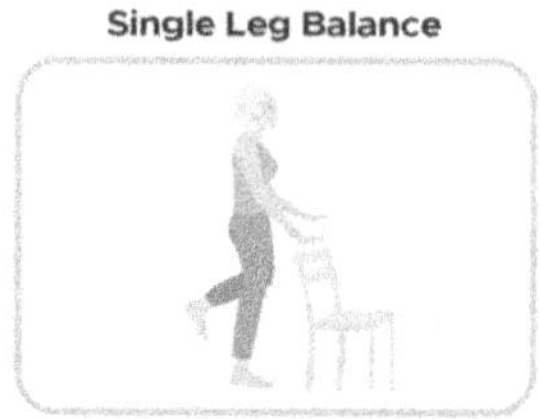

**Single Leg Balance:** Stand behind the chair with your hands lightly resting on the backrest and your feet hip-width apart. Lift your left foot off the ground, bending at the knee. Release your hands from the chair and focus on maintaining your balance. Hold the pose for 30-60 seconds, engaging your core and strengthening your leg muscles. Repeat on the other side to improve balance and stability.

These exercises promote flexibility, strength, and relaxation, making them ideal for enhancing overall well-being and posture.

## Day 5 Warm-Up: Energizing Your Body

As you embark on your fitness journey today, let's begin by awakening your body with a series of invigorating warm-up exercises. Picture yourself in a serene setting, surrounded by the gentle rustle of leaves and the warmth of the morning sun. Take a deep breath in, and let's get started with our day five warm-ups:

Warm-Ups: Perform as many repetitions as you feel comfortable with.

Shoulder Rolls

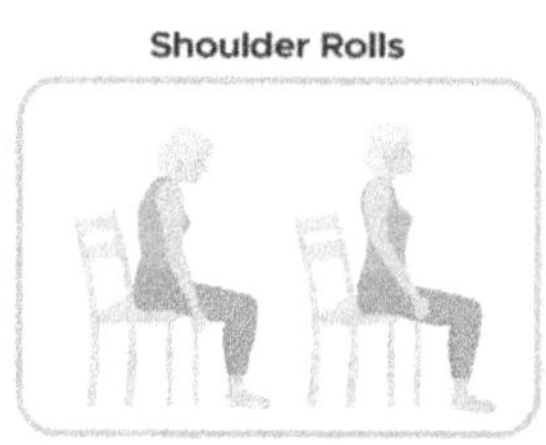

**Shoulder Rolls:** To do shoulder rolls, close your eyes and slowly lift your shoulders up towards your ears while inhaling. Then, roll them back and down while exhaling. Repeat this movement in a clockwise and counterclockwise direction, while being mindful of your breath. This exercise can help to release tension in your shoulders and improve your posture.

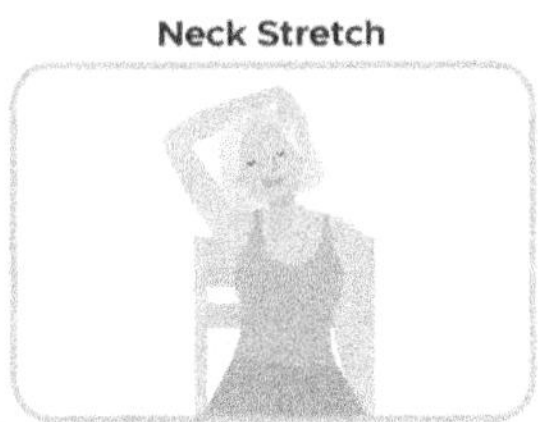

Neck Stretch

**Neck Tilts:** While keeping your back straight, gently tilt your head towards your left shoulder. Hold for two breaths, then return to the center. Repeat on the right side. Perform this twice on each side.

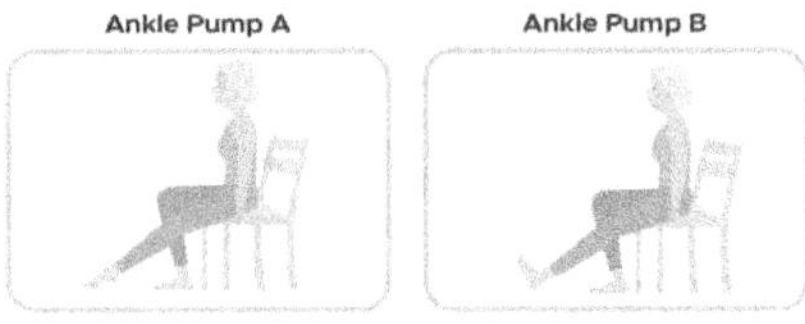

Ankle Pump A    Ankle Pump B

**Ankle Pumps:** Perform ankle pumps by lifting heels and toes alternately, repeating five times. Remember to breathe.

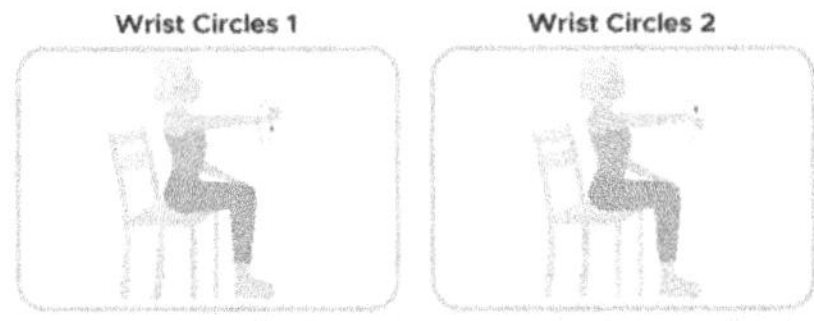

Wrist Circles 1    Wrist Circles 2

**Wrist Circles:** Extend your arms in front with palms facing down. Begin rotating your wrists clockwise for five rotations, then counterclockwise for another five.

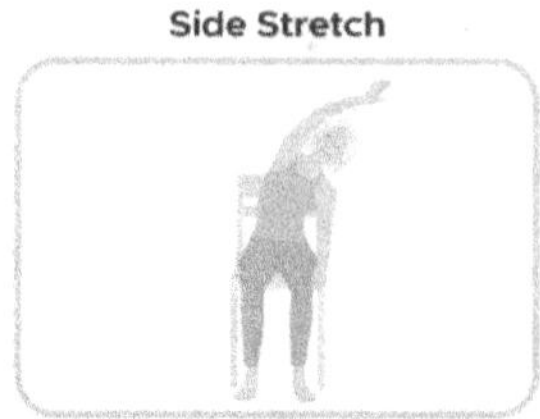



**Side Stretch:** Extend your arms overhead while inhaling. While exhaling, lean to the left side for a gentle stretch. Return to the center while inhaling, then lean to the right while exhaling. Repeat this twice on each side.

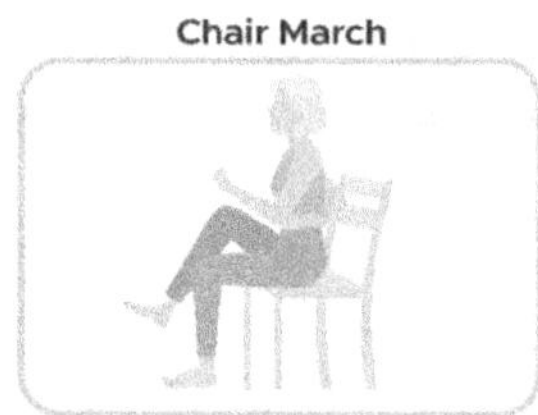



**Chair March:** This can also be done standing next to your chair. Sit up straight with your feet on the floor and arms bent at the elbows. Begin by lifting your right foot and left arm up while pushing your right arm back. Transition to left arm and right foot up as if you were marching. Continue this motion for 3 minutes at a moderate pace.

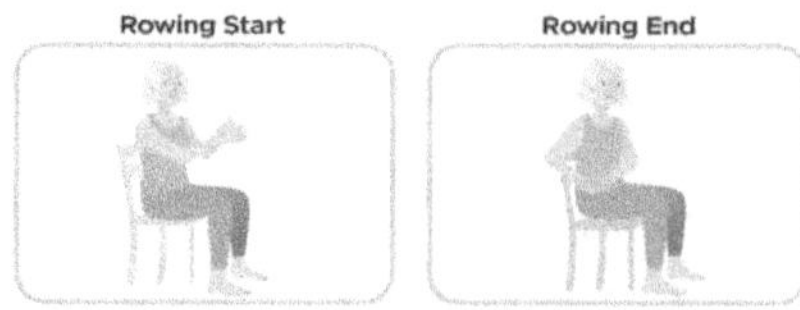



**Seated Rowing:** Start by sitting forward in your chair. Clasp your hands together and stretch them out in front of you to your left side. "Paddle" your hands from front to back at a medium speed as if you are rowing a canoe. Repeat this movement five times, then switch to the right side and repeat. Perform the entire sequence four times.

## Day 5 Main Sequence: Strengthening Your Core and Improving Posture

Now that your body is warmed up let's dive into the main sequence of exercises designed to enhance your posture and strengthen your core muscles.

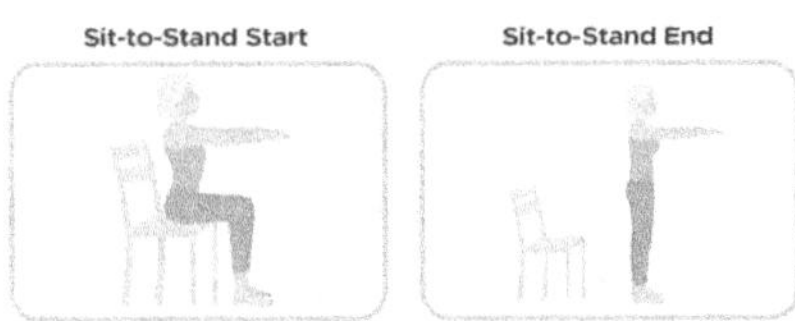


**Sit-to-Stand:** Building Strength and Stability. Imagine yourself seated at the front edge of a sturdy chair, feeling grounded and centered. Your feet are firmly planted on the floor, spaced apart to the width of your hips, ready to embark on this empowering exercise. As you prepare to rise, let's explore the intricacies of the sit-to-stand movement:

Begin by placing your hands on the tops of your thighs or on the chair's armrests, whichever feels more comfortable and supportive for you. With a gentle forward lean, engage your core muscles and push into your hands as you gradually straighten your legs to stand up. Feel the strength coursing through your thighs as you lift yourself upright.

Now, slowly reverse the motion, lowering yourself back down into the seated position with control and grace. Let each movement be deliberate, focusing on the connection between your mind and body as you transition between sitting and standing. Repeat this sequence several times, allowing the rhythm of your breath to guide you through each repetition.

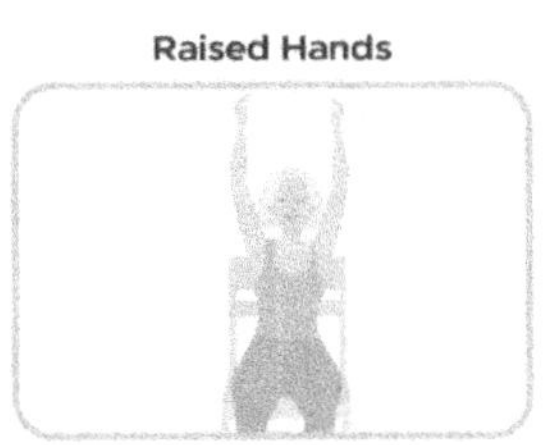

. . .

**Raised Hands Pose:** Reaching for Vitality. Sit comfortably with your back straight and your feet firmly planted on the floor, feeling grounded and rooted. As you inhale deeply, visualize energy flowing through your body, revitalizing every cell. With slow and deliberate movements, raise your arms above your head, aligning them with your ears as much as possible.

Feel the stretch radiating through your shoulders, upper back, and chest as you embrace this moment of expansion and openness. Keep your shoulders relaxed, avoiding any tension or hunching. Hold this pose for a few breaths, allowing yourself to bask in the sensation of upliftment and renewal.

Slowly lower your arms back down to your lap as you exhale, feeling a sense of groundedness and tranquility wash over you. Let each breath be a reminder of your inner strength and resilience, guiding you toward a state of balance and harmony.

**Seated Mountain End**

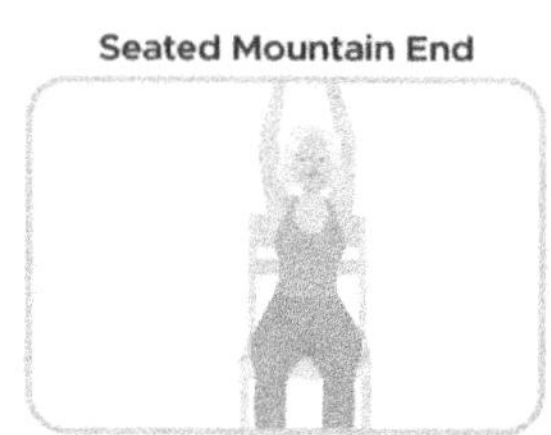

**Seated Mountain Pose:** Sit tall with your feet flat on the floor, aligning your spine and engaging your core muscles. Inhale deeply as you stretch your arms overhead, interlocking your fingers and turning your palms outward. Lift your hands towards the ceiling, aiming to align your head, trunk, and hands. Hold this pose for three to five breaths, feeling the lengthening of your spine and the activation of your core.

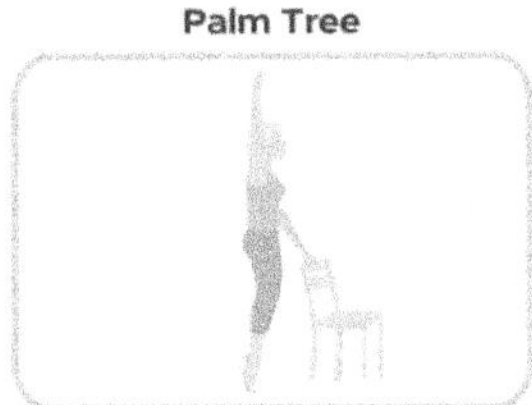



**Palm Tree Pose:** Stand beside your chair, holding onto the backrest with one hand for support. Lift onto the balls of your feet and extend your opposite arm overhead, stretching the side of your body. Return to the starting position and repeat on the other side, feeling a deep stretch along your sides and promoting balance and stability.

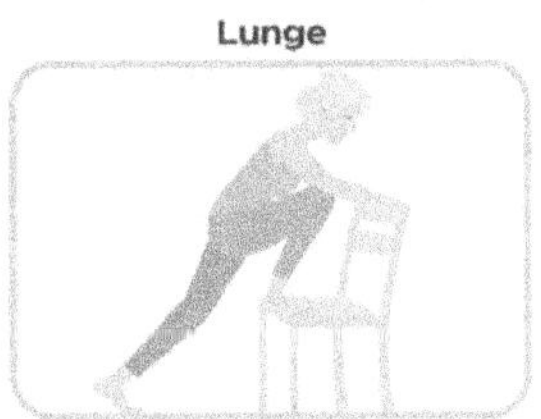



**Lunge:** Stand facing the chair seat with both feet flat on the floor. Grasp the back of the chair with both hands and place one foot on the chair seat. Gently push forward with your other leg, leaning forward to stretch the leg on the chair seat. Hold this position for three breaths before switching sides, targeting your leg muscles and improving flexibility in your hips.

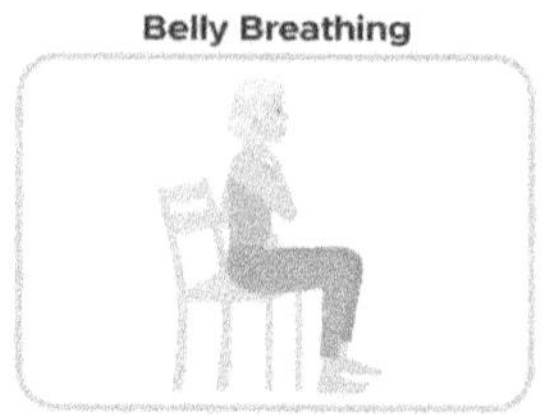



**Seated Deep Breathing:** Nourishing Your Inner Being up tall, embodying a sense of presence and awareness in your body. Place one hand on your belly and the other on your chest, connecting with the rhythm of your breath. As you inhale deeply through your nose, feel your abdomen expand and rise, filling with revitalizing air.

Ensure that your chest remains still, allowing the breath to flow naturally and effortlessly. Exhale slowly through your nose, feeling a sense of release and relaxation wash over you. Repeat this cycle of deep breathing, allowing each inhale to replenish your energy and each exhale to release any tension or stress.

Let the gentle rhythm of your breath anchor you in the present moment, guiding you toward a state of calm and inner peace. With each cycle of breath, feel yourself becoming more grounded and centered, ready to embrace whatever the day may bring.

**Day 6 Warm-Up Routine:** Perform as many repetitions as you feel comfortable with.

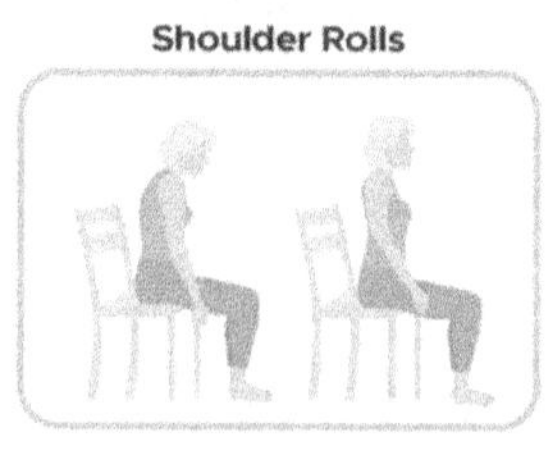

**Shoulder Rolls:** To do shoulder rolls, close your eyes and slowly lift your shoulders up towards your ears while inhaling. Then, roll them back and down while exhaling. Repeat this movement in a clockwise and counterclockwise direction, while being mindful of your breath. This exercise can help to release tension in your shoulders and improve your posture.

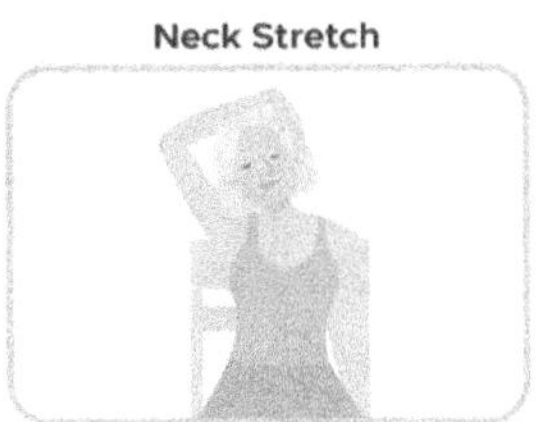



**Neck Tilts:** While keeping your back straight, gently tilt your head towards your left shoulder. Hold for two breaths, then return to the center. Repeat on the right side. Perform this twice on each side.

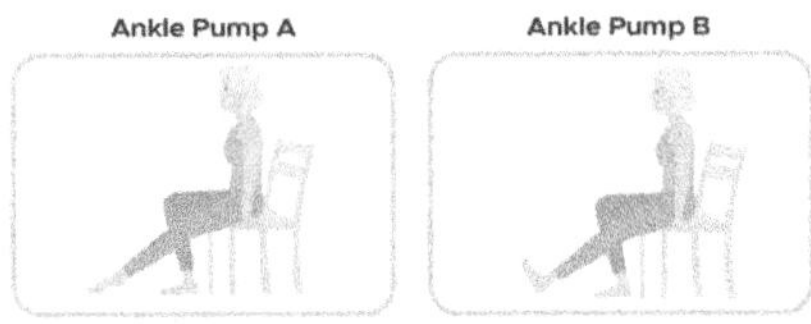



Perform ankle pumps by lifting heels and toes alternately, repeating five times. Remember to breathe.

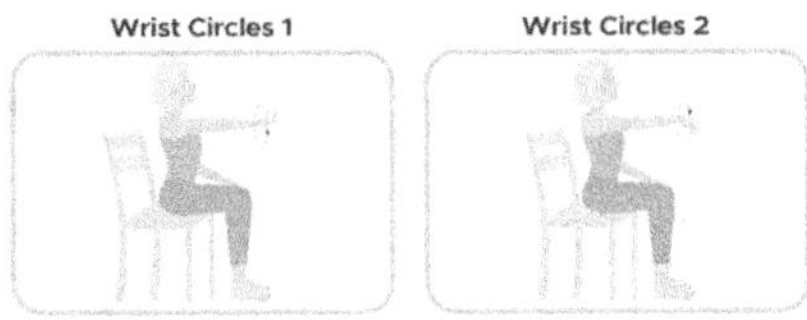



**Wrist Circles:** Extend your arms in front with palms facing down. Begin rotating your wrists clockwise for five rotations, then counter-clockwise for another five.

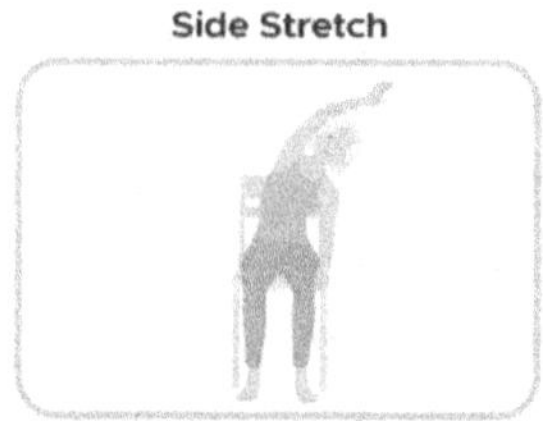

Side Stretch

**Side Stretch:** Extend your arms overhead while inhaling. While exhaling, lean to the left side for a gentle stretch. Return to the center while inhaling, then lean to the right while exhaling. Repeat this twice on each side.

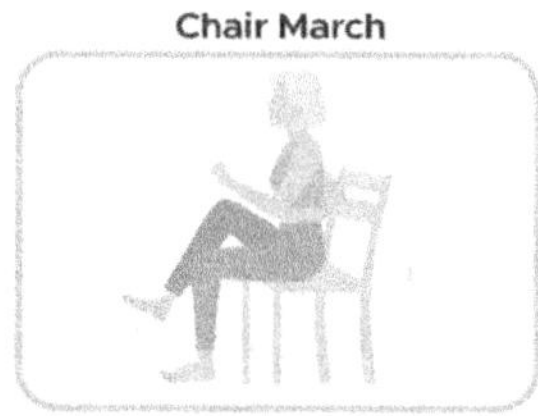

Chair March

**Chair March:** This can also be done standing next to your chair. Sit up straight with your feet on the floor and arms bent at the elbows. Begin by lifting your right foot and left arm up while pushing your right arm back. Transition to left arm and right foot up as if you were marching. Continue this motion for 5-10 minutes at a moderate pace.

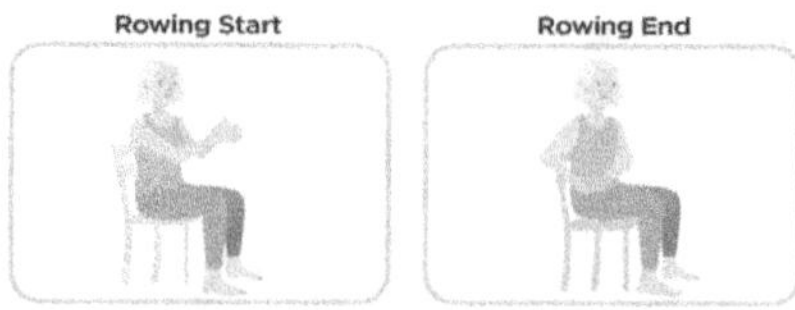

Rowing Start    Rowing End

**Seated Rowing:** Start by sitting forward in your chair. Clasp your hands together and stretch them out in front of you to your left side. "Paddle" your hands from front to back at a medium speed as if you are rowing a canoe. Repeat this movement five times, then switch to the right side and repeat. Perform the entire sequence four times.

**Day 6 Main Sequence:**

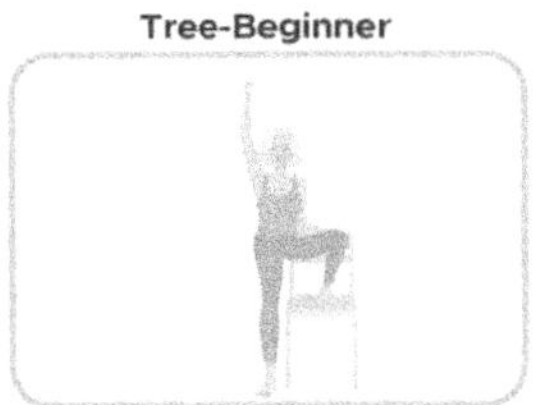



**Balanced Tree Pose:** Stand beside your chair, holding onto the backrest for support. Place your right foot flat on the ground and lift your left foot, placing the sole against the inner thigh or calf of the standing leg. Extend your right arm overhead and hold for several breaths. Repeat on the opposite side.

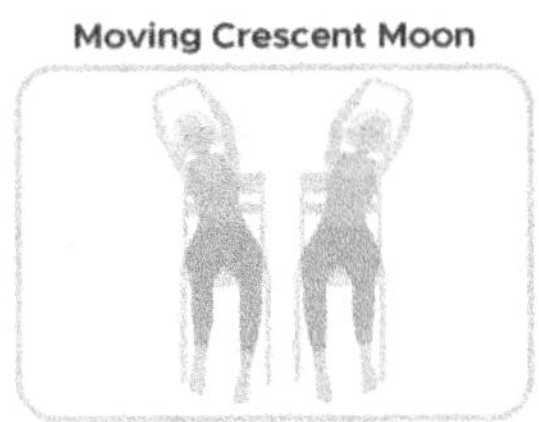



**Moving Crescent Moon Pose:** Sit upright in your chair, clasping your hands together and stretching your arms overhead. Lean your body to the right, holding for two breaths, then return to the center. Repeat on the left side. Repeat this stretch sequence several times.

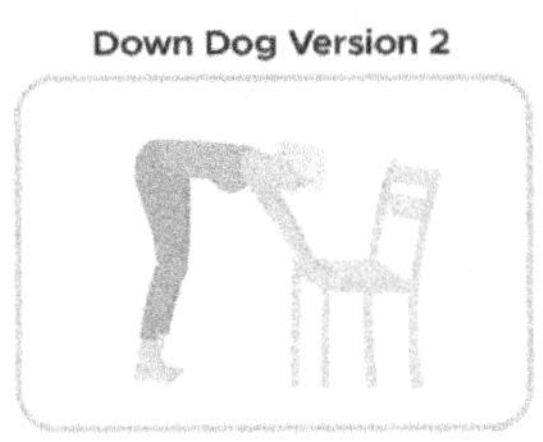



**Down Dog Cheair Pose:** Stand facing the front of your chair at arm's length. Spread your fingers wide and place them on the seat of the chair.

Step your feet back until your arms are straight, forming an inverted "V" with your body. Hold this pose for 3-5 breaths. Repeat as desired.

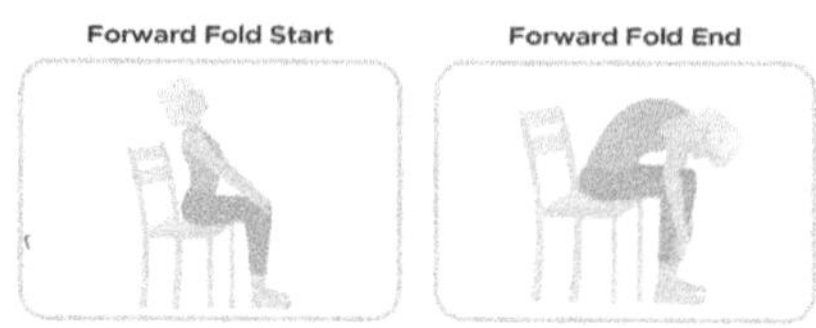


**Forward Fold:** Sit at the edge of your chair with your feet flat on the ground. Inhale and bend forward from the waist, reaching towards the floor. Hold onto your ankles and slide your buttocks forward on the chair to stretch your legs. Hold the pose, breathing deeply, for 3-5 breaths. Repeat twice.

## Day 7 Rest Day/ Mindful Breathing

### Relaxing Breathing Techniques for Focus and Peace

**Box Breathing:** Inhale gently through your nose, counting to four. Hold your breath for four counts. Exhale slowly through your mouth for four counts. Hold the exhale for another count of four. Repeat this rhythmic cycle 5-10 times to promote calmness and center your mind.

**Ocean Breath:** Find a comfortable seated position with relaxed posture. Inhale deeply through your nose, maintaining closed lips. Exhale through your nose while gently constricting the back of your throat, creating a soft, soothing sound reminiscent of ocean waves. Practice this tranquil technique 5-10 times to enhance focus and mindfulness.

**Belly Breathing:** Sit comfortably with a straight back. Place one hand on your chest and the other on your belly. Inhale deeply through your nose, allowing your belly to expand while keeping your chest still. Exhale slowly through your mouth, drawing your belly inward. Continue for a few minutes, focusing on the gentle rise and fall of your belly to promote relaxation and ease stress.

**Ocean Sounding Breath:** Sit upright with relaxed shoulders. Inhale slowly through your nose, then exhale through your nose while gently constricting the back of your throat. Aim for a soft, whisper-like sound during both inhalation and exhalation, similar to fogging a mirror. Repeat this calming exercise ten times to cultivate a sense of peace and clarity.

**Humming Breath (Calming, Stress Relief):** Close your eyes and take a slow, deep breath through your nose. Exhale slowly through your mouth while humming softly. Repeat this soothing practice 5-10 times to calm your mind and release tension.

**Day 8 Warm-Up Routine:** Warm-Ups: Perform as many repetitions as you feel comfortable with.

Shoulder Rolls

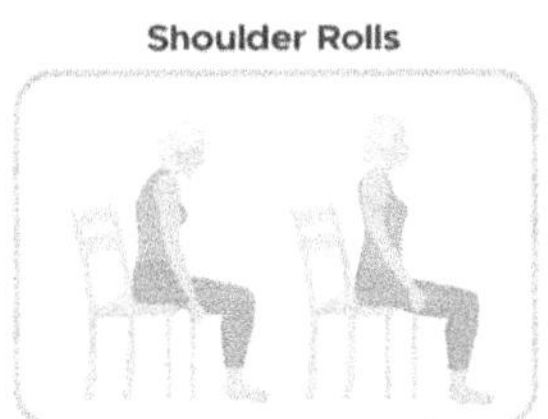

**Shoulder Rolls:** To do shoulder rolls, close your eyes and slowly lift your shoulders up towards your ears while inhaling. Then, roll them back and down while exhaling. Repeat this movement in a clockwise and counterclockwise direction, while being mindful of your breath. This exercise can help to release tension in your shoulders and improve your posture.

Neck Stretch

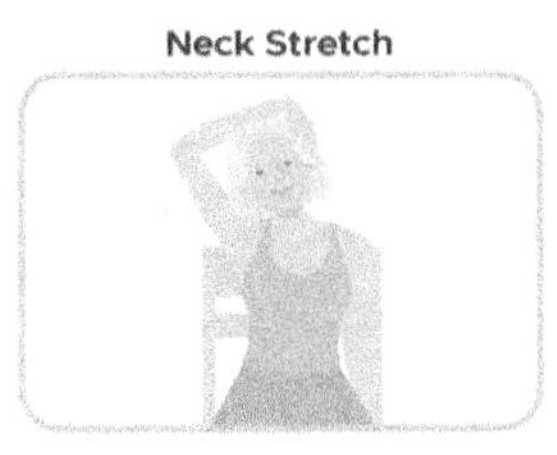

**Neck Tilts:** While keeping your back straight, gently tilt your head towards your left shoulder. Hold for two breaths, then return to the center. Repeat on the right side. Perform this twice on each side.

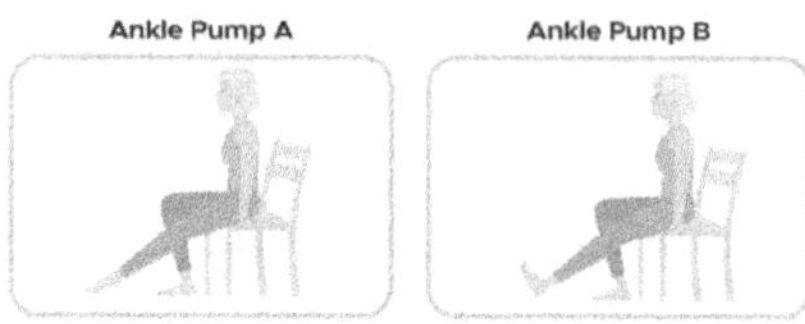


**Ankle Pumps:** Perform ankle pumps by lifting heels and toes alternately, repeating five times. Remember to breathe.

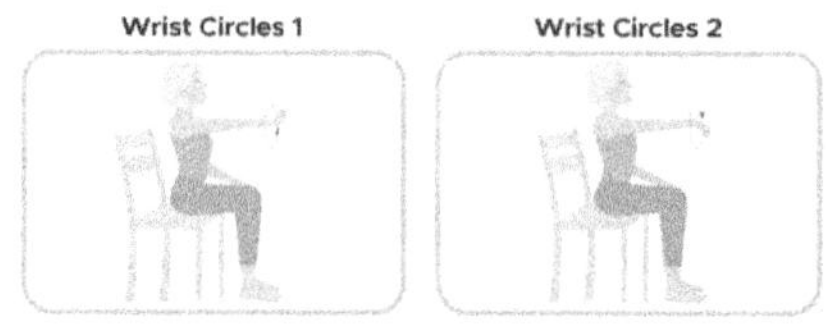


**Wrist Circles:** Extend your arms in front with palms facing down. Begin rotating your wrists clockwise for five rotations, then counterclockwise for another five.

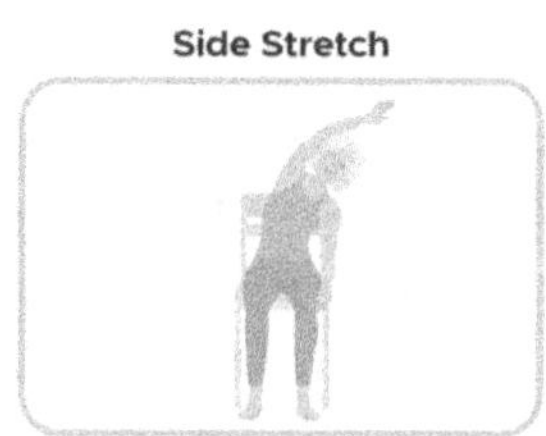


**Side Stretch:** Extend your arms overhead while inhaling. While exhaling, lean to the left side for a gentle stretch. Return to the center while inhaling, then lean to the right while exhaling. Repeat this twice on each side.

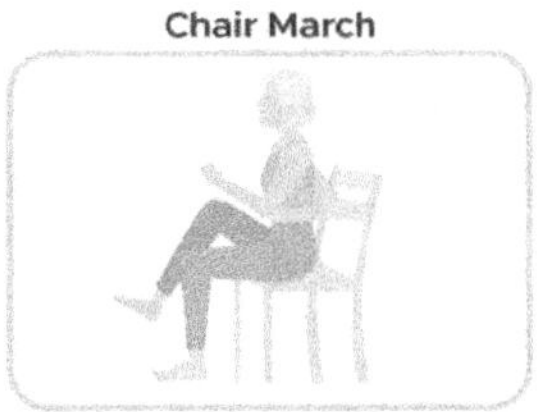

Chair March

**Chair March:** This can also be done standing next to your chair. Sit up straight with your feet on the floor and arms bent at the elbows. Begin by lifting your right foot and left arm up while pushing your right arm back. Transition to left arm and right foot up as if you were marching. Continue this motion for 3 minutes at a moderate pace.

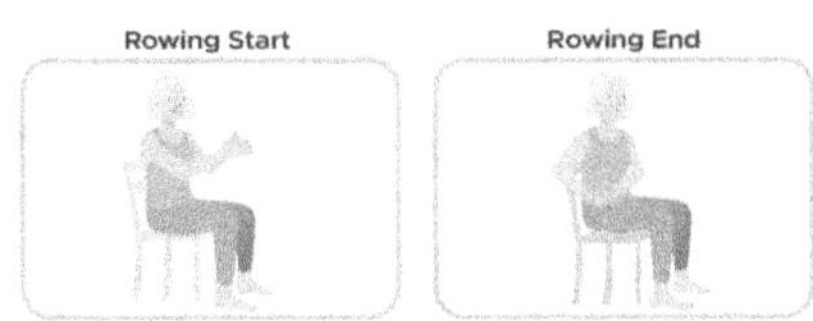

Rowing Start    Rowing End

**Seated Rowing:** Start by sitting forward in your chair. Clasp your hands together and stretch them out in front of you to your left side. "Paddle" your hands from front to back at a medium speed as if you are rowing a canoe. Repeat this movement five times, then switch to the right side and repeat. Perform the entire sequence four times.

**Day 8 Main Sequence:**

**Engaging Chair Yoga Poses for Relaxation and Flexibility**

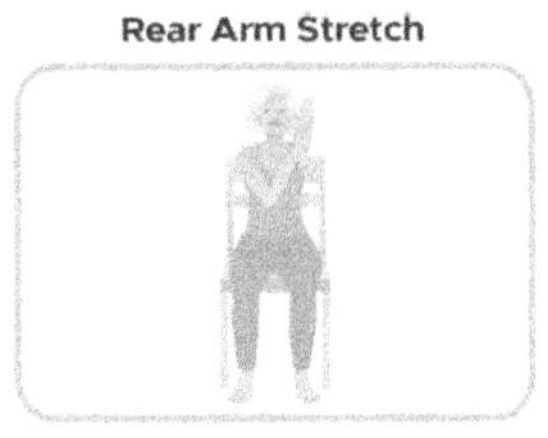

Rear Arm Stretch

**Rear Arm Stretch:** Face forward and reach your right arm back over your right shoulder, attempting to touch your back. Use your opposite hand to gently push below the elbow for a deeper stretch. Hold this position for 10 seconds, then switch sides to release tension in both shoulders and arms.

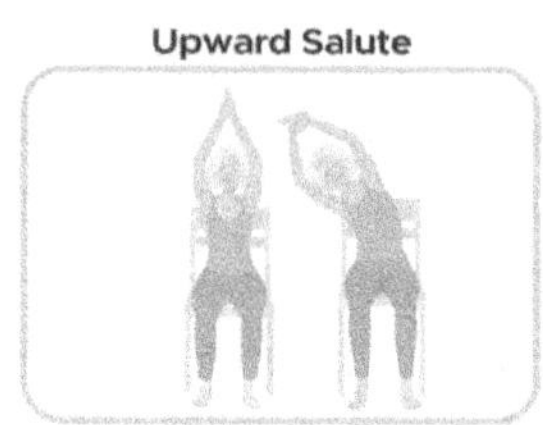



**Upward Salute:** Sit upright with your feet flat on the floor. Inhale and extend your arms overhead, palms facing each other. Gaze straight ahead or slightly upwards without straining your neck. Hold this uplifting pose for three to five breaths, then gently lower your arms on the exhale, feeling a sense of rejuvenation and calm.

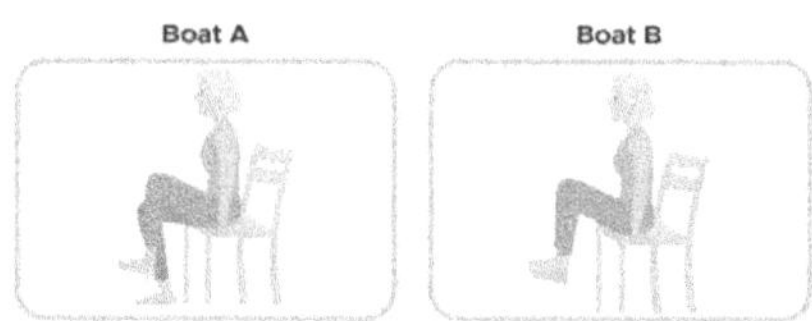



**Seated Boat Pose (Version 1):** Sit comfortably in the middle of your chair with feet flat on the floor. Grasp the sides of the chair for support. Lean back slightly and lift one foot off the floor at a time, drawing your knees toward your chest. Hold this engaging pose for several breaths before gently lowering your feet. Repeat four times, alternating which leg you lift first each time, to strengthen your core and improve balance.

**Leg Forward**

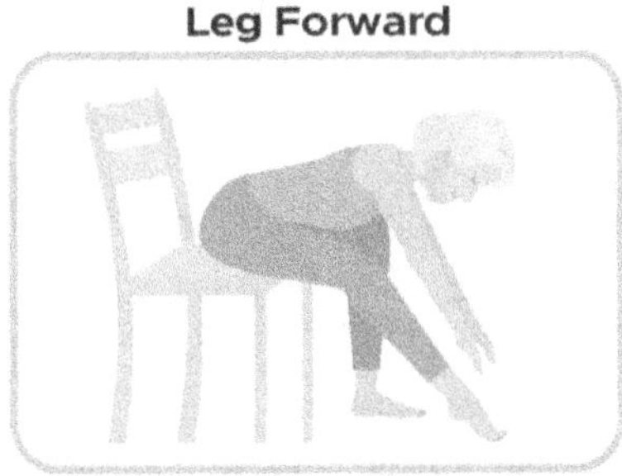

**Leg Forward Bends:** Sit straight with your feet flat on the ground. Inhale deeply and extend one leg straight out in front of you while keeping the other foot firmly on the floor. Exhale and bend forward, reaching towards your extended leg and aiming to touch your toes. Hold this invigorating stretch for three to five breaths, then switch legs to balance your stretch on both sides.

**Pigeon**

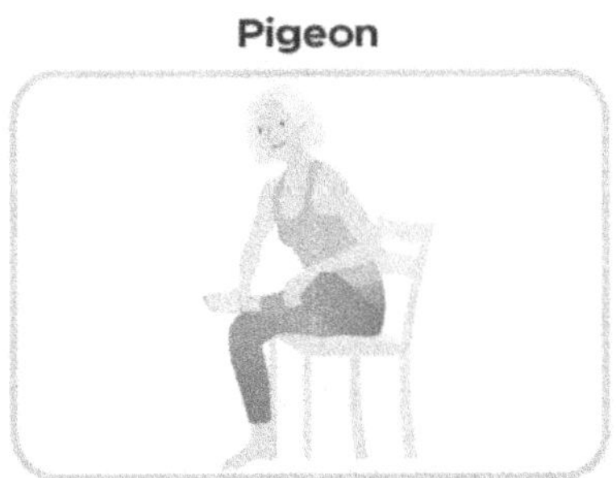

**Pigeon Pose:** Sit upright with both feet flat on the floor. Lift your left ankle and place it over your right thigh, forming a figure-four shape. Point your left knee outward as much as comfortable. For a deeper stretch, gently press down on the left knee. Hold this soothing position for several breaths, then switch sides to ensure a balanced stretch.

**Day 9 Warm-Up Routine:** Warm-Ups: Perform as many repetitions as you feel comfortable with.

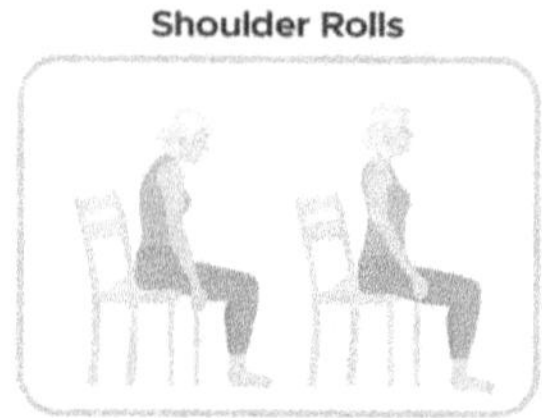



**Shoulder Rolls:** To do shoulder rolls, close your eyes and slowly lift your shoulders up towards your ears while inhaling. Then, roll them back and down while exhaling. Repeat this movement in a clockwise and counterclockwise direction, while being mindful of your breath. This exercise can help to release tension in your shoulders and improve your posture.

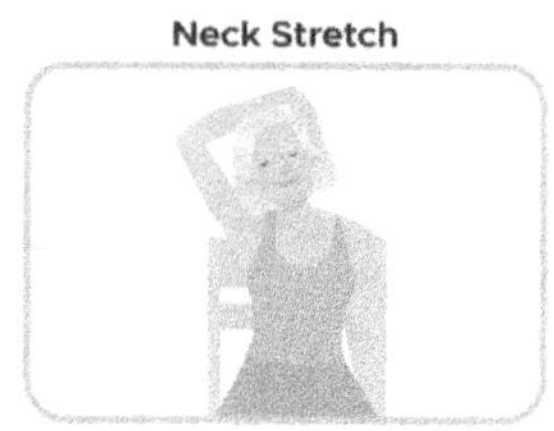



**Neck Tilts:** While keeping your back straight, gently tilt your head towards your left shoulder. Hold for two breaths, then return to the center. Repeat on the right side. Perform this twice on each side.

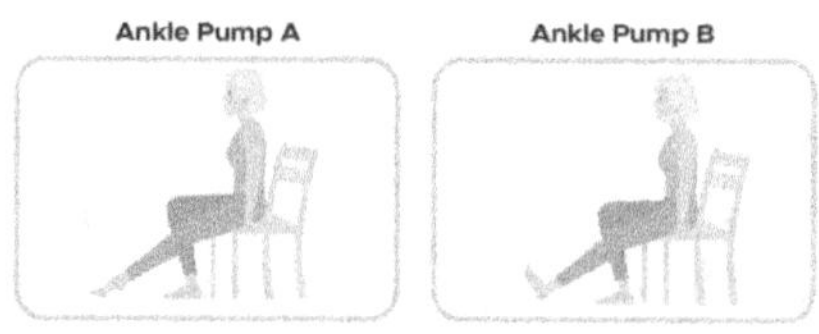



**Ankle Pumps:** Perform ankle pumps by lifting heels and toes alternately, repeating five times. Remember to breathe.

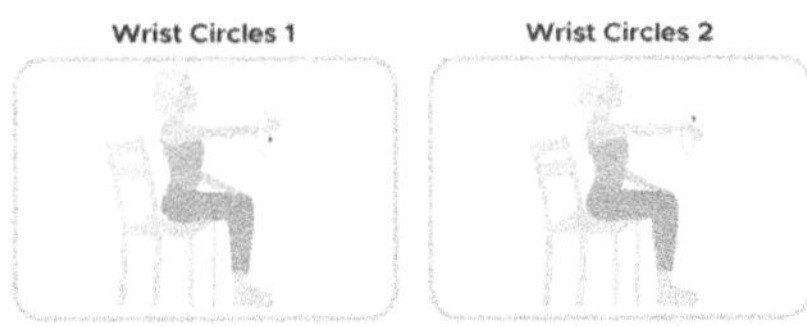


**Wrist Circles:** Extend your arms in front with palms facing down. Begin rotating your wrists clockwise for five rotations, then counter-clockwise for another five.

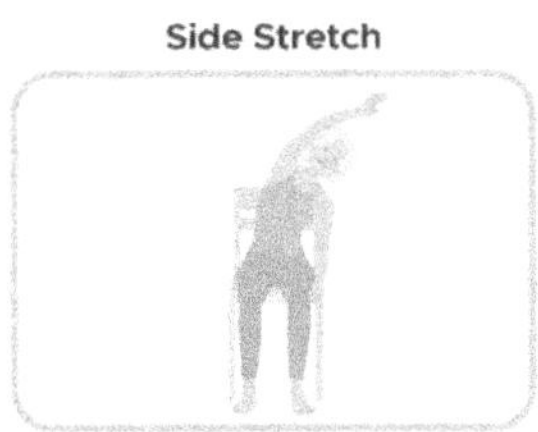


**Side Stretch:** Extend your arms overhead while inhaling. While exhaling, lean to the left side for a gentle stretch. Return to the center while inhaling, then lean to the right while exhaling. Repeat this twice on each side.

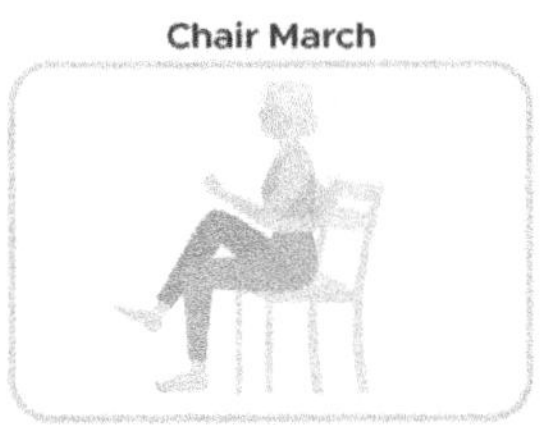


**Chair March:** This can also be done standing next to your chair. Sit up straight with your feet on the floor and arms bent at the elbows. Begin by lifting your right foot and left arm up while pushing your right arm back. Transition to left arm and right foot up as if you were marching. Continue this motion for 3 minutes at a moderate pace.

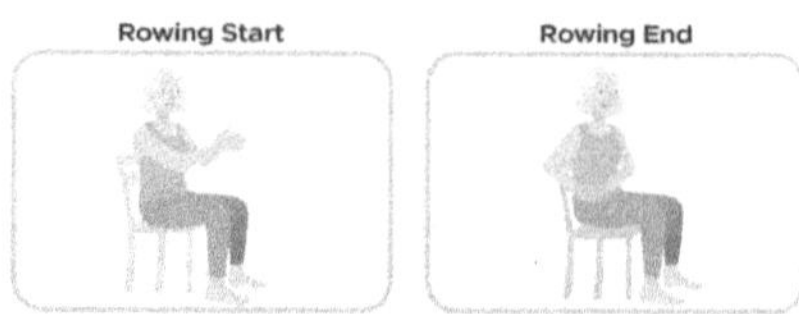


**Seated Rowing:** Start by sitting forward in your chair. Clasp your hands together and stretch them out in front of you to your left side. "Paddle" your hands from front to back at a medium speed as if you are rowing a canoe. Repeat this movement five times, then switch to the right side and repeat. Perform the entire sequence four times.

## Day 9 Main Sequence: Energizing Chair Yoga Poses

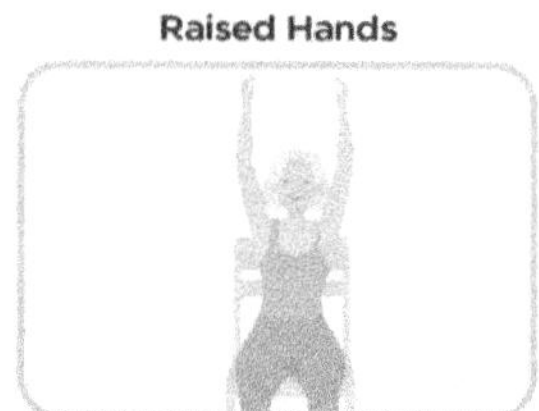


**Elevated Hands Pose:** Begin by sitting comfortably with your back straight and feet firmly on the floor. As you slowly inhale, raise your arms above your head, aligning them with your ears. Keep your shoulders relaxed and avoid hunching. Hold this pose for three to five breaths, then gently lower your hands back to your lap as you exhale, feeling the energy flow through your body.

*Note: For the next three poses, aim to transition from Warrior 1 to Warrior 2 to Reverse Warrior. However, practicing them separately at first may be helpful.*

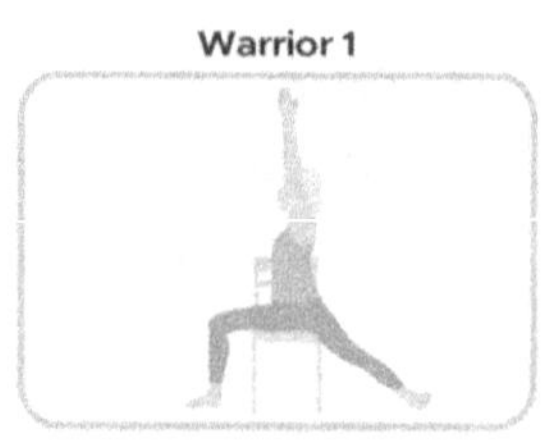

**Warrior 1:** Sit sideways on the chair with your right leg in front and your left leg extended behind you, straightening it as much as possible. As you inhale, raise your arms towards the ceiling, keeping your torso aligned over your right leg. Hold this empowering pose for several breaths, feeling the strength of Warrior 1.

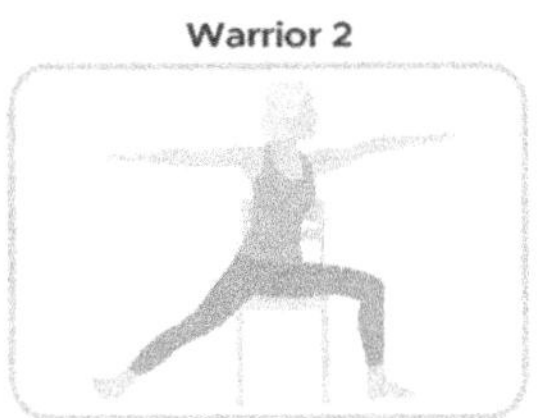

Warrior 2

**Warrior 2:** Turn your torso to face the front of the chair and extend your arms out to the sides, palms facing down. Take deep, calming breaths, inhaling and exhaling three times. Embrace the stability and focus of Warrior 2.

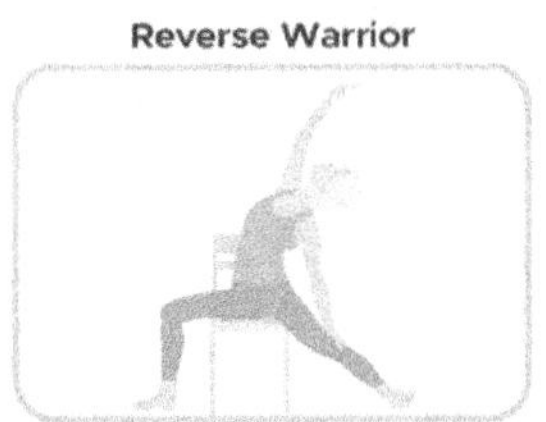

Reverse Warrior

**Reverse Warrior:** Slowly glide your left hand down towards your left foot while lifting your right hand upwards, bending it slightly over your head to open up your chest and side. Hold this rejuvenating pose for four deep breaths, enjoying the stretch and expansion of Reverse Warrior. If these poses feel strenuous, take a moment to rest before continuing.

**Day 10 Rest/Breathing Exercises:**

**Relaxing Breathing Techniques for Focus and Peace**

**Box Breathing:** Inhale gently through your nose, counting to four. Hold your breath for four counts. Exhale slowly through your mouth for four counts. Hold the exhale for another count of four. Repeat this rhythmic cycle 5-10 times to promote calmness and center your mind.

**Ocean Breath:** Find a comfortable seated position with relaxed posture. Inhale deeply through your nose, maintaining closed lips. Exhale through your nose while gently constricting the back of your throat, creating a soft, soothing sound reminiscent of ocean waves. Practice this tranquil technique 5-10 times to enhance focus and mindfulness.

**Belly Breathing:** Sit comfortably with a straight back. Place one hand on your chest and the other on your belly. Inhale deeply through your nose, allowing your belly to expand while keeping your chest still. Exhale slowly through your mouth, drawing your belly inward. Continue for a few minutes, focusing on the gentle rise and fall of your belly to promote relaxation and ease stress.

**Ocean Sounding Breath:** Sit upright with relaxed shoulders. Inhale slowly through your nose, then exhale through your nose while gently constricting the back of your throat. Aim for a soft, whisper-like sound during both inhalation and exhalation, similar to fogging a mirror. Repeat this calming exercise ten times to cultivate a sense of peace and clarity.

**Humming Breath (Calming, Stress Relief):** Close your eyes and take a slow, deep breath through your nose. Exhale slowly through your mouth while humming softly. Repeat this soothing practice 5-10 times to calm your mind and release tension.

**Day 11 Warm-Up Routine:** Warm-Ups: Perform as many repetitions as you feel comfortable with.

**Shoulder Rolls**

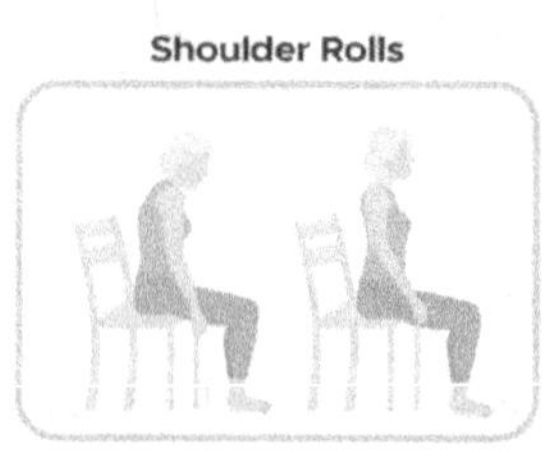

**Shoulder Rolls:** To do shoulder rolls, close your eyes and slowly lift your shoulders up towards your ears while inhaling. Then, roll them back and down while exhaling. Repeat this movement in a clockwise and counterclockwise direction, while being mindful of your breath. This exercise can help to release tension in your shoulders and improve your posture.

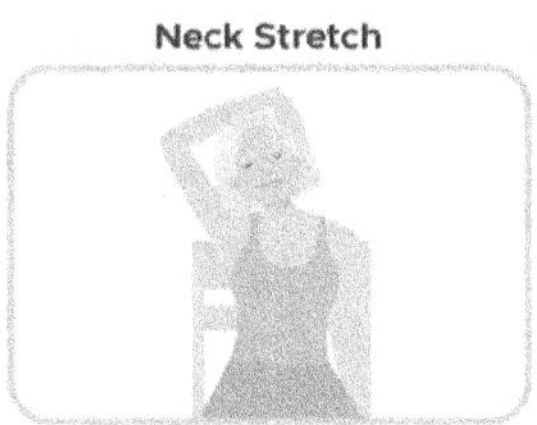

Neck Stretch

**Neck Tilts:** While keeping your back straight, gently tilt your head towards your left shoulder. Hold for two breaths, then return to the center. Repeat on the right side. Perform this twice on each side.

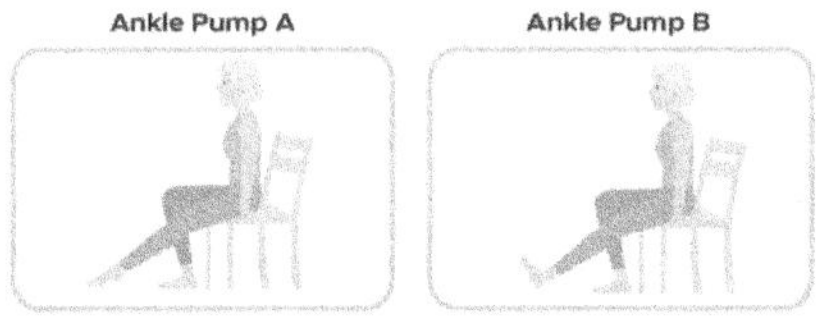

Ankle Pump A          Ankle Pump B

**Ankle Pumps:** Perform ankle pumps by lifting heels and toes alternately, repeating five times. Remember to breathe.

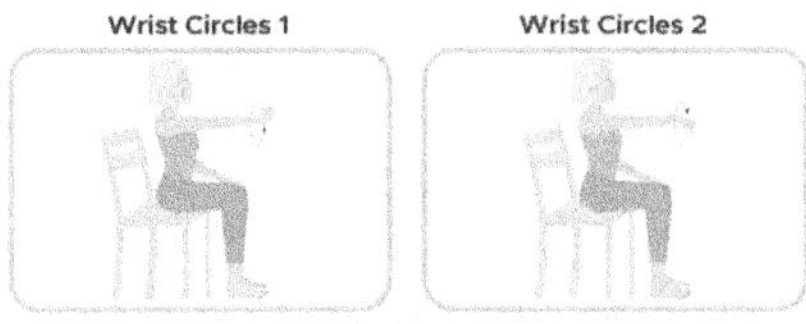

Wrist Circles 1          Wrist Circles 2

**Wrist Circles:** Extend your arms in front with palms facing down. Begin rotating your wrists clockwise for five rotations, then counterclockwise for another five.

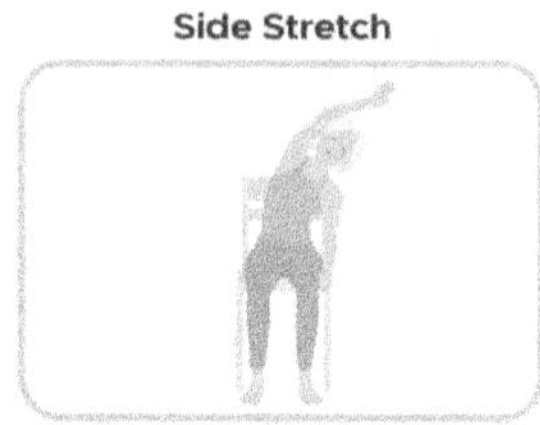


**Side Stretch:** Extend your arms overhead while inhaling. While exhaling, lean to the left side for a gentle stretch. Return to the center while inhaling, then lean to the right while exhaling. Repeat this twice on each side.

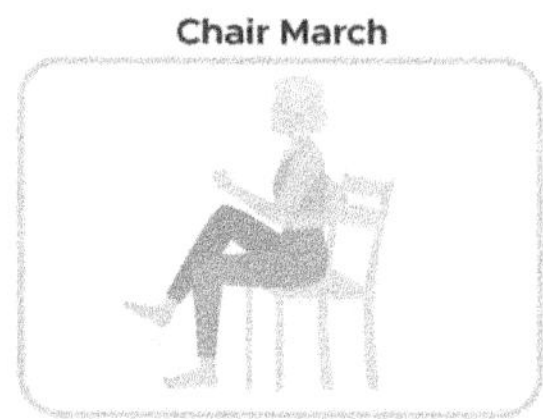


**Chair March:** This can also be done standing next to your chair. Sit up straight with your feet on the floor and arms bent at the elbows. Begin by lifting your right foot and left arm up while pushing your right arm back. Transition to left arm and right foot up as if you were marching. Continue this motion for 3 minutes at a moderate pace.

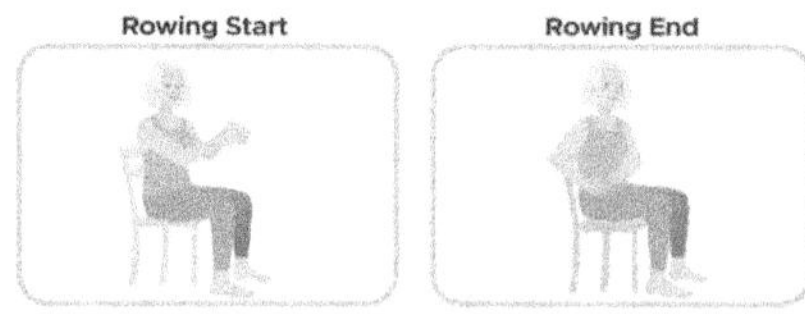


**Seated Rowing:** Start by sitting forward in your chair. Clasp your hands together and stretch them out in front of you to your left side. "Paddle" your hands from front to back at a medium speed as if you are rowing a canoe. Repeat this movement five times, then switch to the right side and repeat. Perform the entire sequence four times.

## Day 11 Main Sequence: Dynamic Chair Yoga Flow

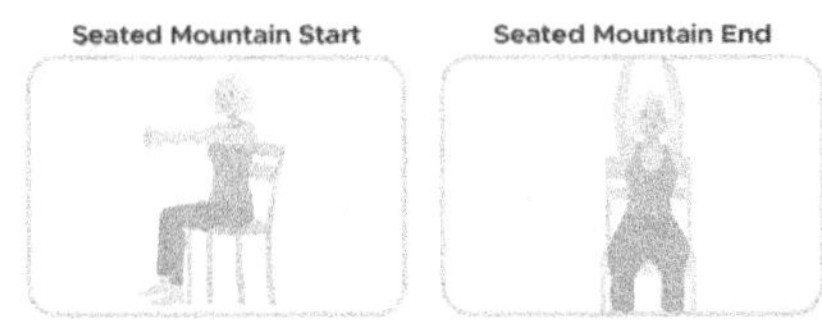


**Seated Mountain:** Start by sitting straight with your feet flat on the floor. Inhale deeply as you stretch your arms out, interlocking your fingers and turning your palms outward. Raise your hands above your head with your palms facing the ceiling, aligning your head, trunk, and hands. Hold this uplifting pose for 3-5 breaths, feeling the length and strength in your spine.

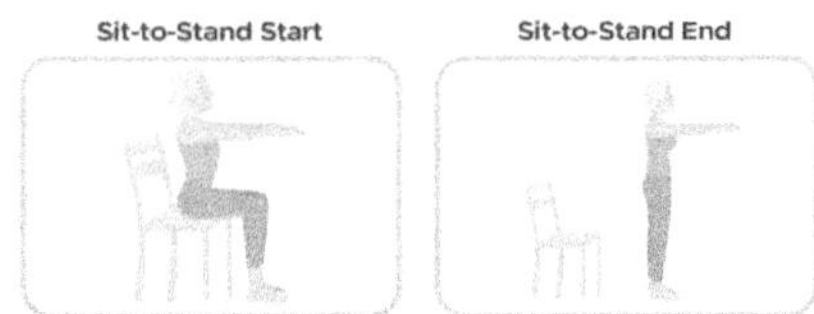


**Sit-to-Stand:** Move to the front edge of your chair with your feet flat on the floor, hip-width apart. Place your hands on the tops of your thighs or the chair's armrests. Lean forward slightly and push into your hands while straightening your legs to stand up. Slowly reverse the movement to sit back down. Repeat this energizing exercise 5-10 times rapidly, building strength and mobility.

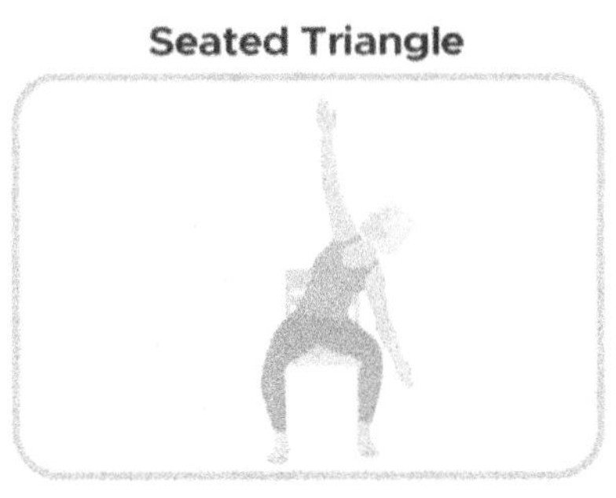

**Seated Triangle:** Sit upright towards the edge of your chair with your legs spread shoulder-width apart. Extend your arms out to the sides like an airplane, palms facing downwards. Hinge at the waist and lean to the right, bringing your right hand towards your right ankle while your left arm points upwards. Breathe deeply and hold this expansive pose for several breaths before transitioning to the other side.

**Single Leg Balance**

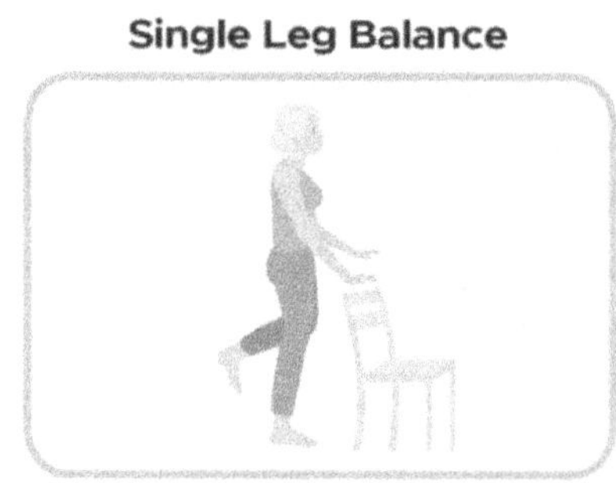

**Single Leg Balance:** Stand behind the chair with your hands loosely on the backrest and your feet flat. Lift your left foot off the ground, bending at the knee. Release the chair and focus on your balance, holding this steady pose for 5-10 seconds. Repeat on the other side, enhancing your stability and coordination.

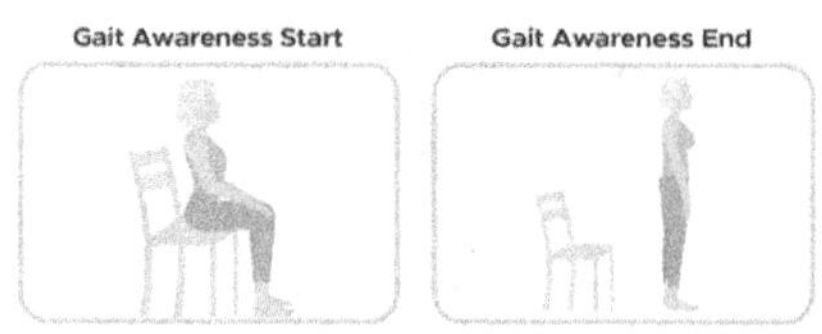


**Gait Awareness Pose:** Begin seated with your hands on your thighs. Stand up just in front of the chair and slowly lift your right knee towards your chest. Step the right foot forward, placing it down heel first. Shift your weight onto the right foot, lift the left foot, and step it forward in the same deliberate manner. Continue this mindful walking for several steps, then turn around and repeat in the opposite direction, improving your coordination and balance.

**Day 12 Warm-Up Routine:** Warm-Ups: Perform as many repetitions as you feel comfortable with.

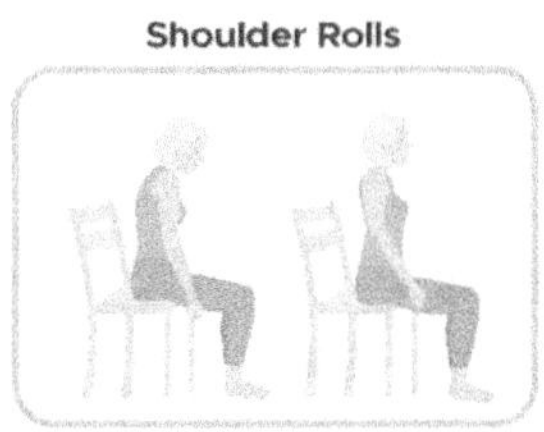

Shoulder Rolls

**Shoulder Rolls:** To do shoulder rolls, close your eyes and slowly lift your shoulders up towards your ears while inhaling. Then, roll them back and down while exhaling. Repeat this movement in a clockwise and counterclockwise direction, while being mindful of your breath. This exercise can help to release tension in your shoulders and improve your posture.

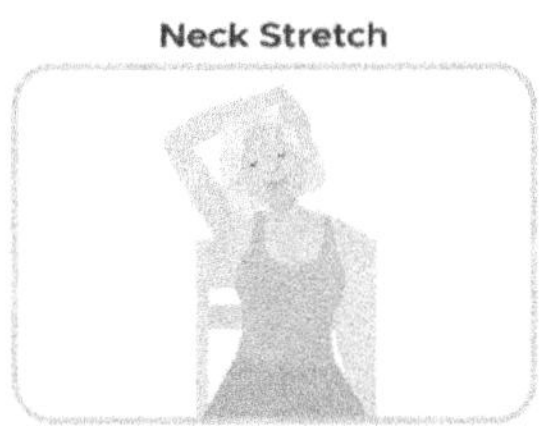

Neck Stretch

**Neck Tilts:** While keeping your back straight, gently tilt your head towards your left shoulder. Hold for two breaths, then return to the center. Repeat on the right side. Perform this twice on each side.

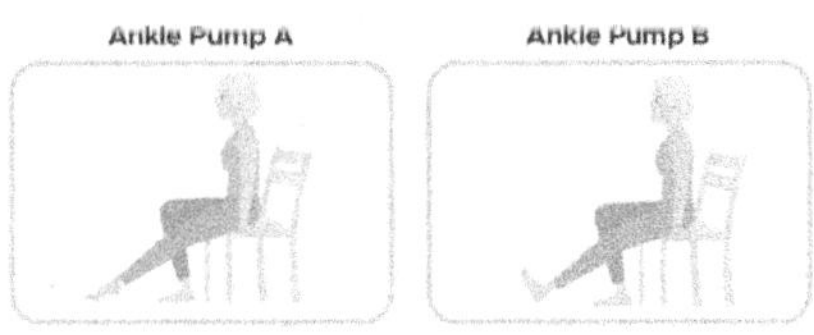

Ankle Pump A          Ankle Pump B

**Ankle Pumps:** Perform ankle pumps by lifting heels and toes alternately, repeating five times. Remember to breathe.

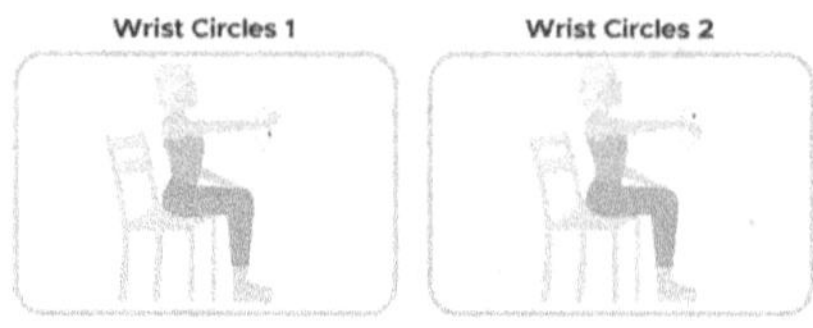

**Wrist Circles:** Extend your arms in front with palms facing down. Begin rotating your wrists clockwise for five rotations, then counter-clockwise for another five.

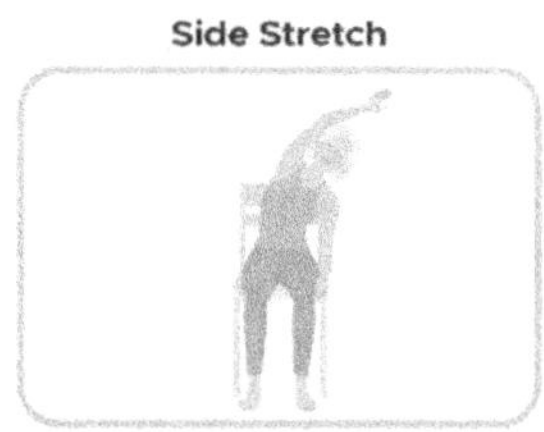

**Side Stretch:** Extend your arms overhead while inhaling. While exhaling, lean to the left side for a gentle stretch. Return to the center while inhaling, then lean to the right while exhaling. Repeat this twice on each side.

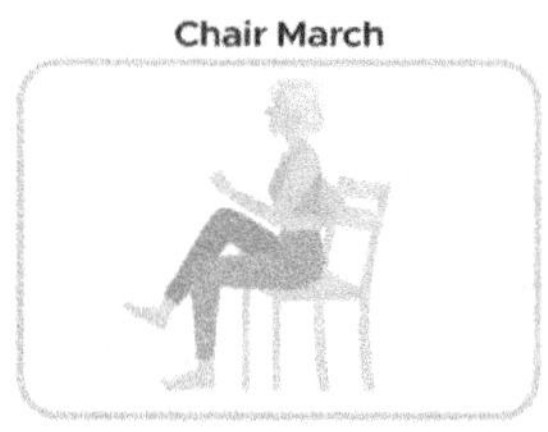

**Chair March:** This can also be done standing next to your chair. Sit up straight with your feet on the floor and arms bent at the elbows. Begin by lifting your right foot and left arm up while pushing your right arm back. Transition to left arm and right foot up as if you were marching. Continue this motion for 3 minutes at a moderate pace.

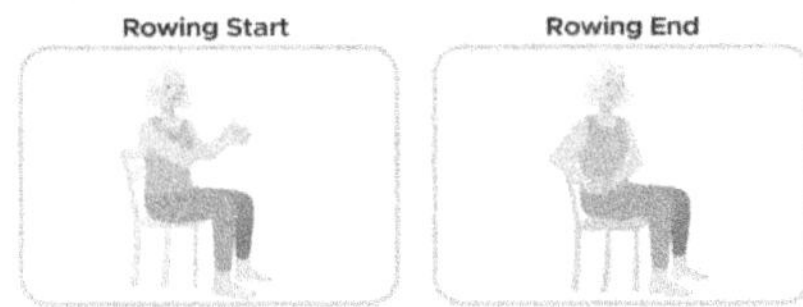



**Seated Rowing:** Start by sitting forward in your chair. Clasp your hands together and stretch them out in front of you to your left side. "Paddle" your hands from front to back at a medium speed as if you are rowing a canoe. Repeat this movement five times, then switch to the right side and repeat. Perform the entire sequence four times.

**Day 12 Main Sequence: Flowing Chair Yoga**

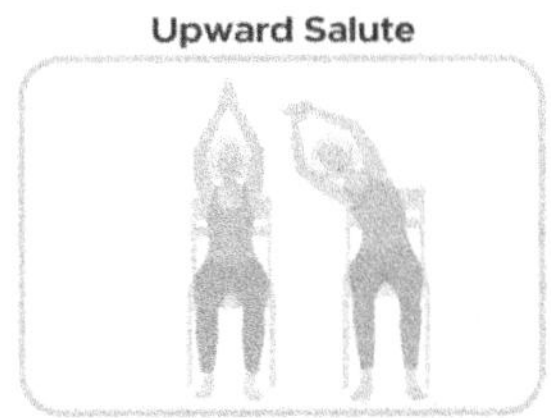



**Upward Salute:** Begin by sitting upright with your feet firmly grounded on the floor. Inhale deeply as you extend your arms overhead, palms facing each other. Keep your gaze forward without straining your neck. Hold this uplifting position for three to five breaths, then gracefully lower your arms on the exhale, feeling a sense of calm and openness.

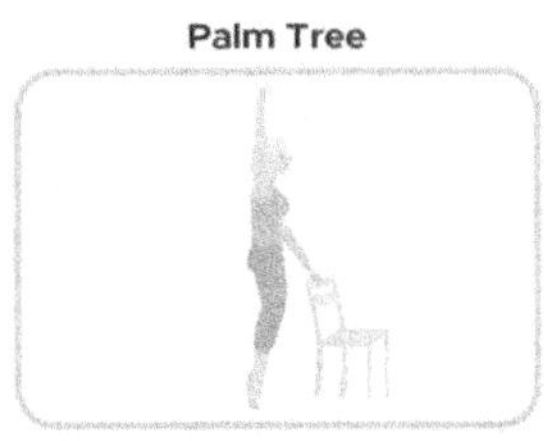



**Palm Tree Pose:** Stand facing the back of the chair, holding onto the backrest with your left hand. Rise onto the balls of your feet, extending your right arm overhead to create a beautiful stretch along the side of your body. Return your hand to the chair and flatten your feet back on the ground. Enjoy the sensation of reaching tall and balanced.

**Foot to Seat**

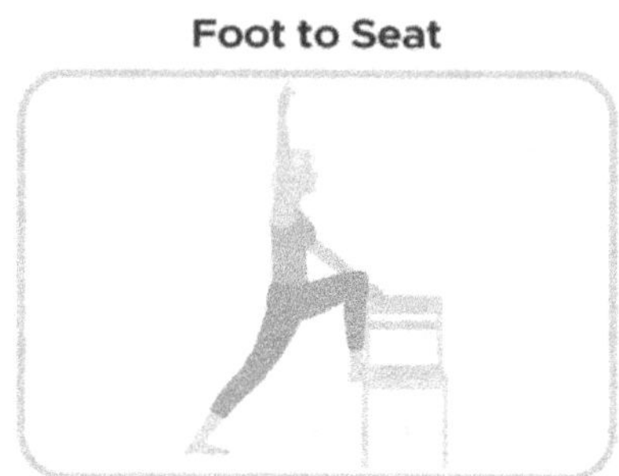

**Foot-to-Seat Pose:** Position yourself beside the chair, about two steps away, and place your right hand on the backrest. Step your left foot onto the seat while extending your left arm overhead, fingers stretched out towards the sky. Hold for three deep breaths, savoring the stretch along your side. Switch sides, grasping the chair with your left hand and stepping your right foot onto the seat, extending your right arm overhead.

**Hero**

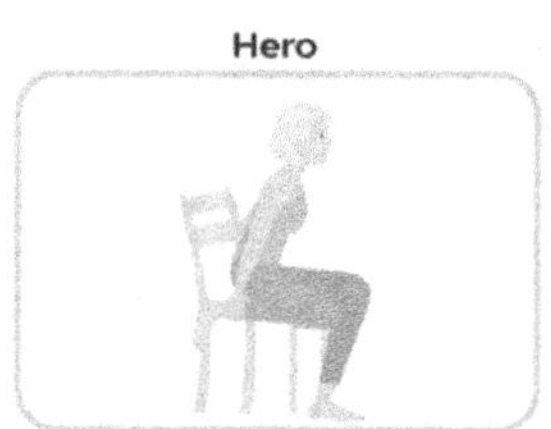

**Hero's Pose:** Slide to the front edge of the seat and extend your left leg backward, keeping the knee bent. Ensure your bent knee points downward and the foot rests comfortably against the side of the chair. Hold this grounding pose for three to five breaths, breathing deeply each time. Return to a neutral position and repeat with the opposite leg, feeling the strength and stability in your posture.

Standing Reverse Warrior

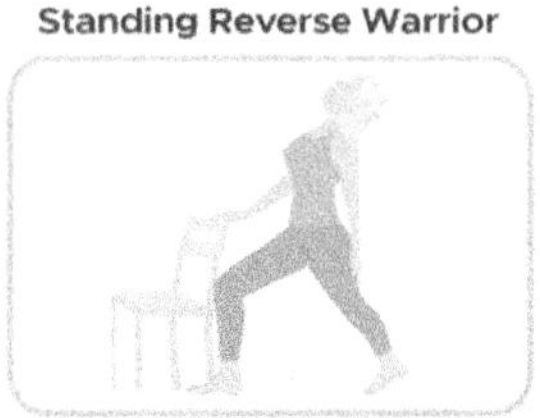

**Standing Reverse Warrior:** Stand behind the chair with your left hand resting on the backrest and both feet slightly under the chair. Slide your right foot back, bending your left knee until it's almost parallel to the floor. Extend your right arm out behind you, feeling the powerful stretch in your body. Hold the pose for 10 seconds, then repeat on the opposite side, experiencing the energy and balance of this warrior stance.

## Day 13 Rest Day/ Mindful Breathing

### Relaxing Breathing Techniques for Focus and Peace

**Box Breathing:** Inhale gently through your nose, counting to four. Hold your breath for four counts. Exhale slowly through your mouth for four counts. Hold the exhale for another count of four. Repeat this rhythmic cycle 5-10 times to promote calmness and center your mind.

**Ocean Breath:** Find a comfortable seated position with relaxed posture. Inhale deeply through your nose, maintaining closed lips. Exhale through your nose while gently constricting the back of your throat, creating a soft, soothing sound reminiscent of ocean waves. Practice this tranquil technique 5-10 times to enhance focus and mindfulness.

**Belly Breathing:** Sit comfortably with a straight back. Place one hand on your chest and the other on your belly. Inhale deeply through your nose, allowing your belly to expand while keeping your chest still. Exhale slowly through your mouth, drawing your belly inward. Continue for a few minutes, focusing on the gentle rise and fall of your belly to promote relaxation and ease stress.

**Ocean Sounding Breath:** Sit upright with relaxed shoulders. Inhale slowly through your nose, then exhale through your nose while gently constricting the back of your throat. Aim for a soft, whisper-like sound during both inhalation and exhalation, similar to fogging a mirror. Repeat this calming exercise ten times to cultivate a sense of peace and clarity.

**Humming Breath (Calming, Stress Relief):** Close your eyes and take a slow, deep breath through your nose. Exhale slowly through your mouth while humming softly. Repeat this soothing practice 5-10 times to calm your mind and release tension.

**Day 14 Warm-Up Routine:** Warm-Ups: Perform as many repetitions as you feel comfortable with.

**Shoulder Rolls**

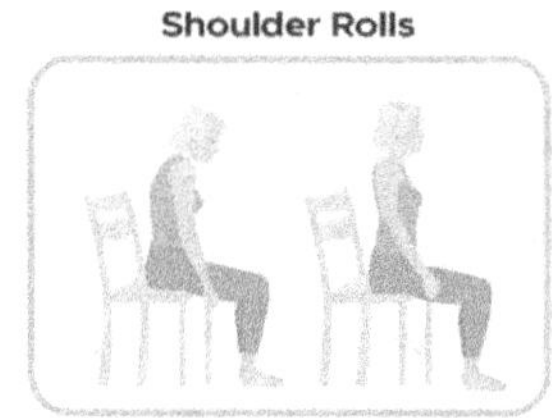

**Shoulder Rolls:** To do shoulder rolls, close your eyes and slowly lift your shoulders up towards your ears while inhaling. Then, roll them back and down while exhaling. Repeat this movement in a clockwise and counterclockwise direction, while being mindful of your breath. This exercise can help to release tension in your shoulders and improve your posture.

**Neck Stretch**

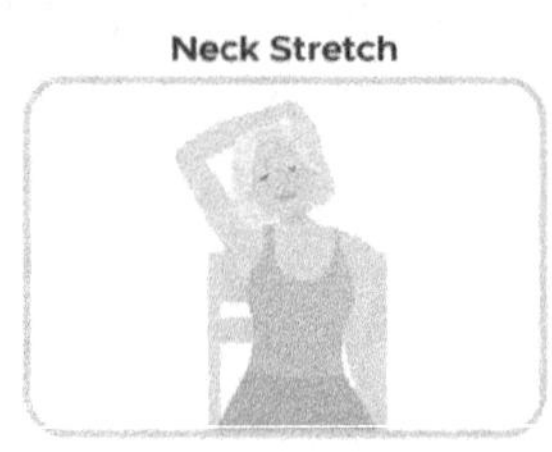

**Neck Tilts:** While keeping your back straight, gently tilt your head towards your left shoulder. Hold for two breaths, then return to the center. Repeat on the right side. Perform this twice on each side.

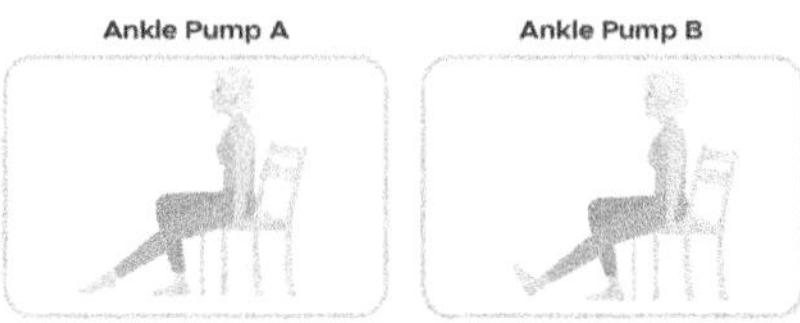


**Ankle Pumps:** Perform ankle pumps by lifting heels and toes alternately, repeating five times. Remember to breathe.

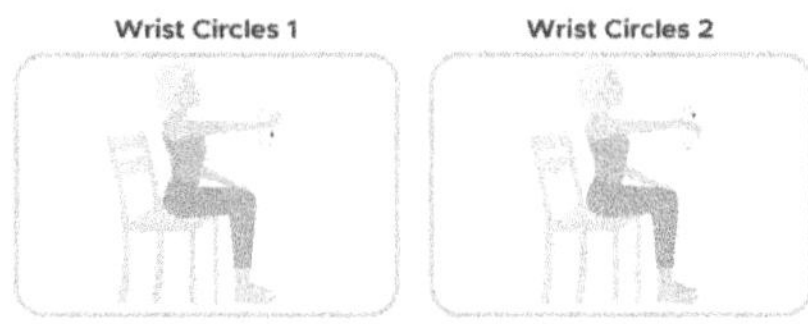


**Wrist Circles:** Extend your arms in front with palms facing down. Begin rotating your wrists clockwise for five rotations, then counterclockwise for another five.

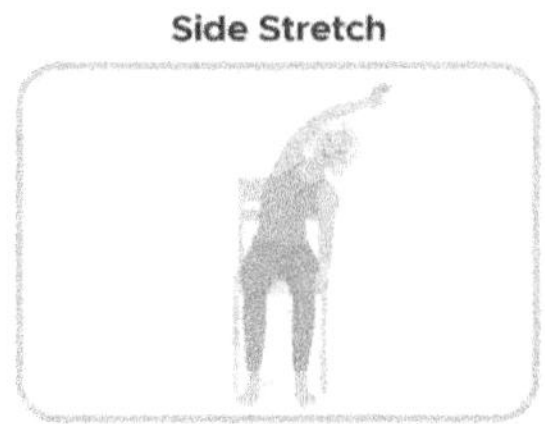


**Side Stretch:** Extend your arms overhead while inhaling. While exhaling, lean to the left side for a gentle stretch. Return to the center while inhaling, then lean to the right while exhaling. Repeat this twice on each side.

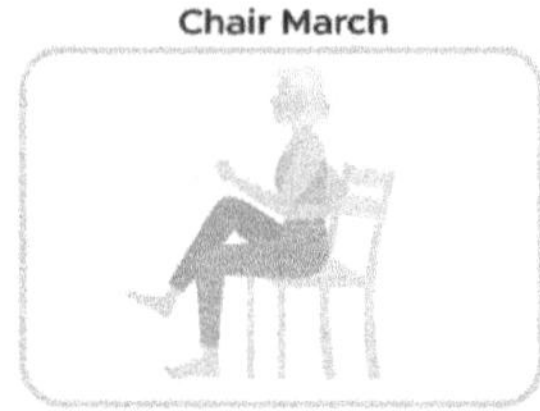

Chair March

**Chair March:** This can also be done standing next to your chair. Sit up straight with your feet on the floor and arms bent at the elbows. Begin by lifting your right foot and left arm up while pushing your right arm back. Transition to left arm and right foot up as if you were marching. Continue this motion for 3 minutes at a moderate pace.

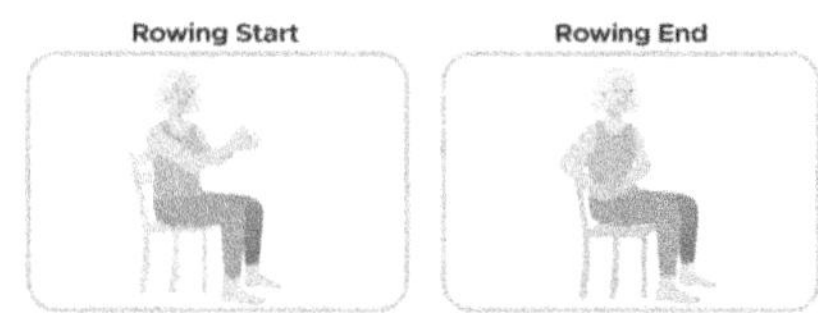

Rowing Start     Rowing End

**Seated Rowing:** Start by sitting forward in your chair. Clasp your hands together and stretch them out in front of you to your left side. "Paddle" your hands from front to back at a medium speed as if you are rowing a canoe. Repeat this movement five times, then switch to the right side and repeat. Perform the entire sequence four times.

**Day 14 Main Sequence: Revitalize and Stretch**

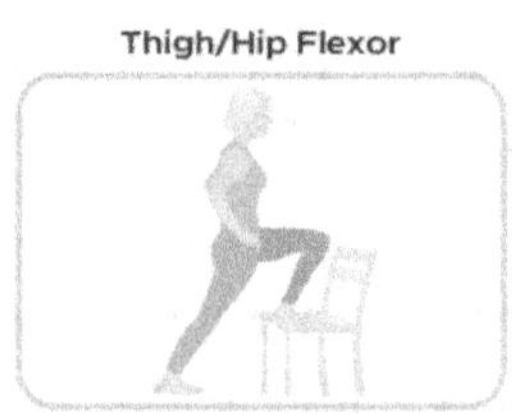

Thigh/Hip Flexor

**Hip Flexor Stretch:** Begin by standing in front of your chair. If you have balance issues, hold onto a second chair for support. Keep your left foot firmly on the floor while extending your right leg and placing the right foot onto the seat of the chair. Keep your spine straight as you gently press your hips forward, feeling a stretch along the front of the extended leg. Breathe deeply and hold for several breaths. Switch sides, placing your right foot on the floor and your left leg on the seat of the chair. Press your hips forward and breathe deeply. Repeat the alternating exercise 3-5 times.

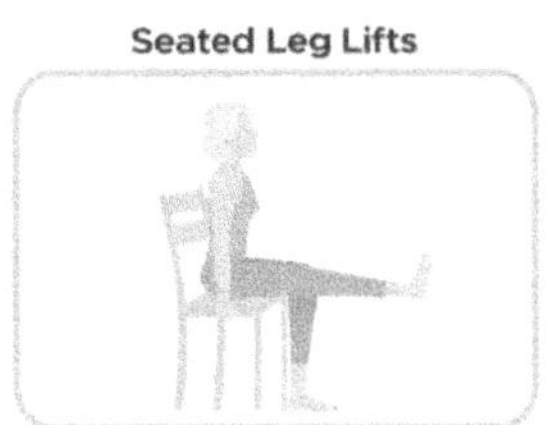

Seated Leg Lifts

**Leg Lifts:** Sit upright in your chair. Extend your right leg straight while keeping the knee straight, and lift the leg to hip height. Hold the leg in the raised position for three breaths, then lower it back to the floor. Repeat with the left leg, extending it straight and lifting it to hip height. Hold for three breaths, feeling the strength and control in your legs.

**Spinal Twist:** Sit upright with your feet flat on the floor. Place your right hand on your left knee. Inhale and lengthen your spine, then exhale and gently twist to the left, using your right hand for slight leverage. Be mindful not to twist too far. Hold for 5-10 breaths, then return to the neutral position and repeat on the opposite side, enjoying the release and flexibility in your spine.

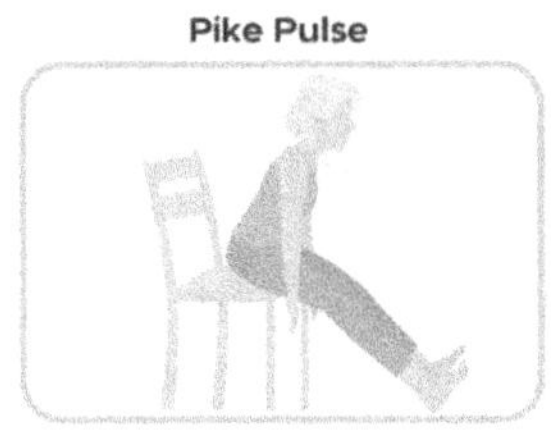

Pike Pulse

**Pike Pulse:** Sit towards the edge of the chair and extend both legs straight out in front of you. Place your hands on the armrests or sides of the chair for support, or keep them beside you. Engage your abs and pulse your legs upwards, lifting them slightly off the ground and back down. Perform ten pulses, keeping your core engaged throughout, and feel the invigorating energy building in your body.

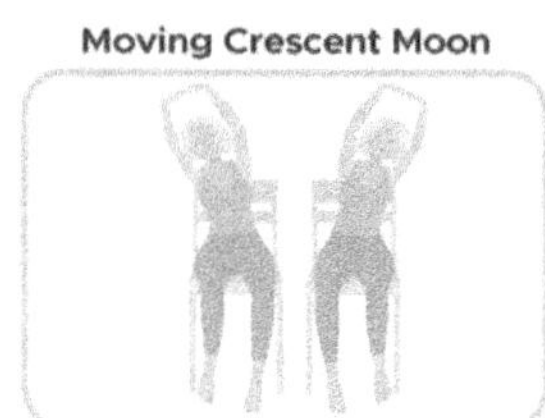


**Moving Crescent Moon Pose:** Sit upright in your chair and stretch both arms overhead, clasping your hands together. Lean your body to the right, holding for two breaths. Inhale while returning to the center, then exhale. Lean your body to the left, holding for two breaths. Inhale while returning to the center, then exhale. Repeat the left-right stretch five times, experiencing the graceful flow and gentle opening of your sides.

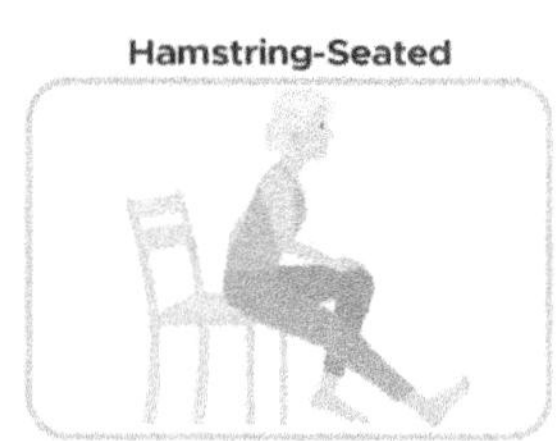


**Seated Hamstring Stretch:** Sit with both feet on the floor and legs at a 90-degree angle. Extend your left leg forward and flex the left foot, keeping the leg straight but not locked at the knee. Hinge at the hips while keeping the back straight, and lean forward until you feel a stretch in the hamstrings. Hold for three breaths. Switch to the other side, extending your right leg forward and flexing the right foot, keeping the leg straight but not locked at the knee. Hinge at the hips and lean forward until you feel a stretch in the hamstrings. Hold for three breaths and return to the center. This pose can also be done from a standing position using the chair as a prop, enhancing flexibility and ease in your hamstrings.

**Day 15 Warm-Up Routine:** Warm-Ups: Perform as many repetitions as you feel comfortable with.

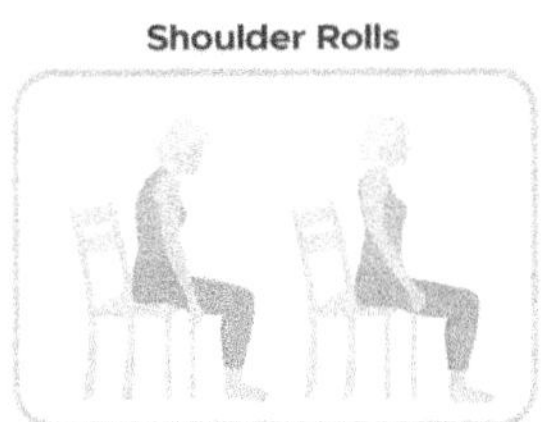

Shoulder Rolls

**Shoulder Rolls:** To do shoulder rolls, close your eyes and slowly lift your shoulders up towards your ears while inhaling. Then, roll them back and down while exhaling. Repeat this movement in a clockwise and counterclockwise direction, while being mindful of your breath. This exercise can help to release tension in your shoulders and improve your posture.

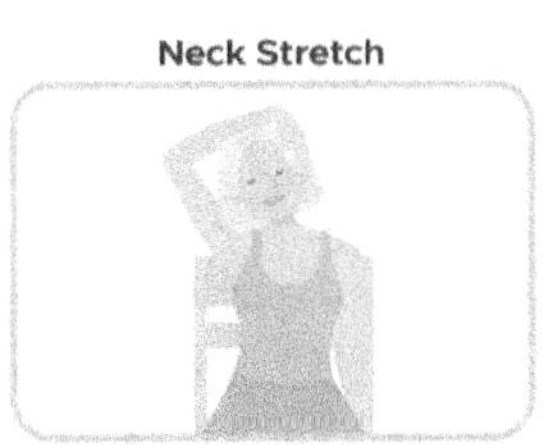

Neck Stretch

**Neck Tilts:** While keeping your back straight, gently tilt your head towards your left shoulder. Hold for two breaths, then return to the center. Repeat on the right side. Perform this twice on each side.

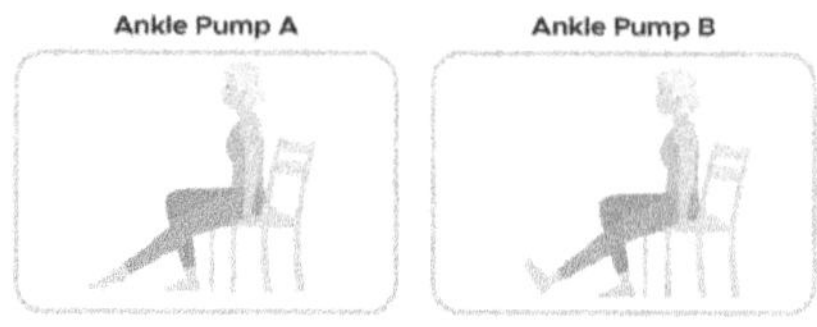

**Ankle Pumps:** Perform ankle pumps by lifting heels and toes alternately, repeating five times. Remember to breathe.

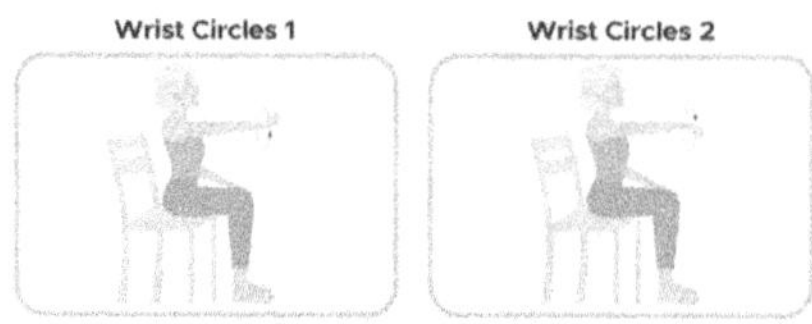

**Wrist Circles:** Extend your arms in front with palms facing down. Begin rotating your wrists clockwise for five rotations, then counterclockwise for another five.

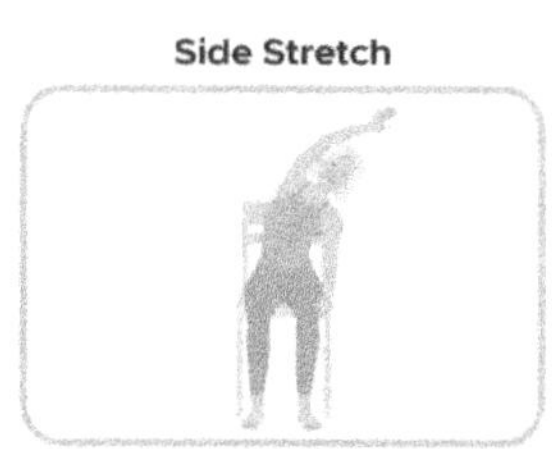

**Side Stretch:** Extend your arms overhead while inhaling. While exhaling, lean to the left side for a gentle stretch. Return to the center while inhaling, then lean to the right while exhaling. Repeat this twice on each side.

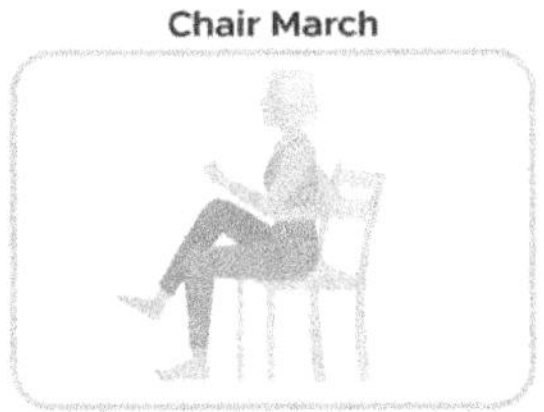

Chair March

**Chair March:** This can also be done standing next to your chair. Sit up straight with your feet on the floor and arms bent at the elbows. Begin by lifting your right foot and left arm up while pushing your right arm back. Transition to left arm and right foot up as if you were marching. Continue this motion for 3 minutes at a moderate pace.

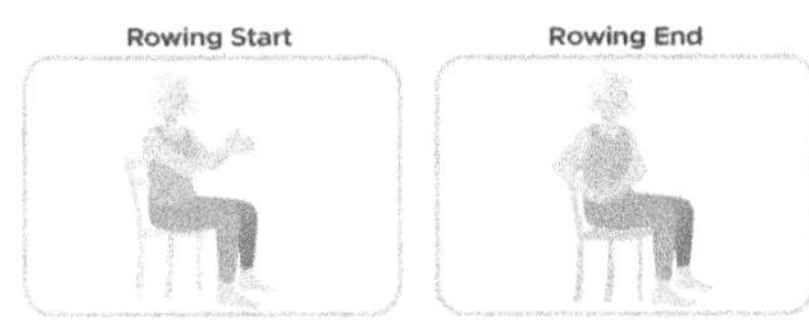

Rowing Start    Rowing End

**Seated Rowing:** Start by sitting forward in your chair. Clasp your hands together and stretch them out in front of you to your left side. "Paddle" your hands from front to back at a medium speed as if you are rowing a canoe. Repeat this movement five times, then switch to the right side and repeat. Perform the entire sequence four times.

**Day 15 Main Sequence: Energize and Stretch**

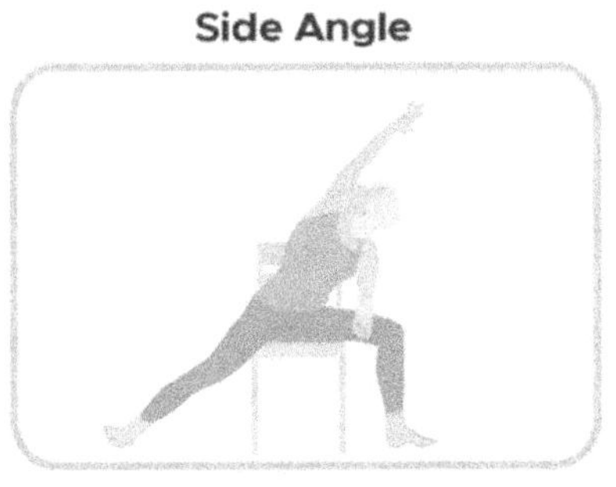

Side Angle

**Side Angle:** Start seated upright with your feet flat on the floor. Place your right hand on your right knee or thigh. Inhale and lift your left arm up towards the ceiling. As you exhale, gently lean to the right, feeling a stretch along the left side of your body. Hold for 5-10 breaths, then return to the starting position. Repeat on the opposite side, enjoying the elongation and balance in your torso.

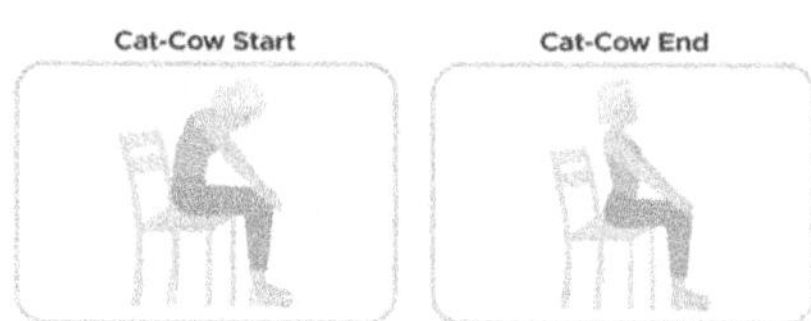


**Cat-Cow Pose:** Seated with your back straight and both feet flat on the floor, place your hands on your knees. Inhale and arch your back, looking up to stretch the front of your neck. Exhale, round your back, tuck in your chin, and stretch the back of your neck. Continue for ten cycles, syncing your movements with your breaths, relishing the gentle wave-like motion along your spine.

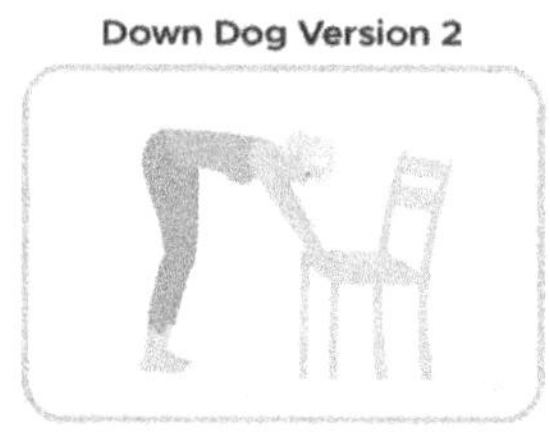


**Down Dog Version 2:** Stand facing the front of the chair, about an arm's length away. Spread your fingers wide and place them on the seat of the chair. Step your feet back until your arms are stretched out straight, forming an inverted V with your body. Push your hips back and up, keeping your feet flat on the floor. Hold this pose for 3-5 breaths, feeling the invigorating stretch in your back and legs. Repeat to enhance flexibility.

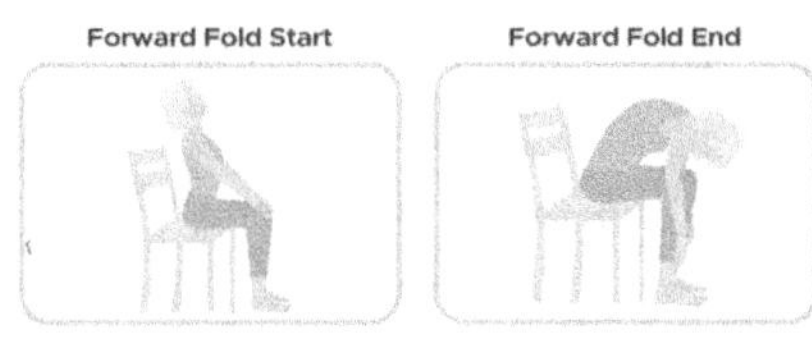


**Forward Fold:** While seated, place your feet flat on the floor and your hands on your knees. Inhale through your nose and lengthen your spine, looking up. Exhale, hinge at the hips, and fold forward, bringing your chest towards your knees. Allow your hands to grasp your lower legs if possible. Hold for 5-10 breaths, feeling the calming release in your back and hamstrings.

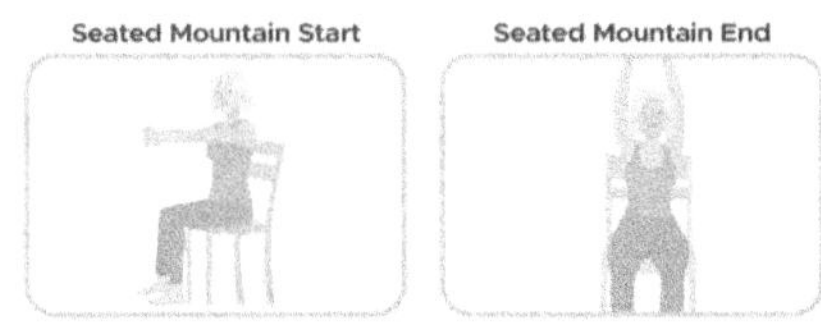


**Seated Mountain:** Sit straight with your feet flat on the floor. Inhale as you stretch your arms out, interlocking your fingers and turning your palms outward. Raise your hands above your head with your palms towards the ceiling, aligning your head, trunk, and hands. Hold for 3-5 breaths, feeling grounded and lengthened from head to toe.

By varying the order and flow of these exercises, you can enjoy a more dynamic and refreshing routine that promotes flexibility, strength, and relaxation.

## Day 16 Rest Day/ Mindful Breathing

### Relaxing Breathing Techniques for Focus and Peace

**Box Breathing:** Inhale gently through your nose, counting to four. Hold your breath for four counts. Exhale slowly through your mouth for four counts. Hold the exhale for another count of four. Repeat this rhythmic cycle 5-10 times to promote calmness and center your mind.

**Ocean Breath:** Find a comfortable seated position with relaxed posture. Inhale deeply through your nose, maintaining closed lips. Exhale through your nose while gently constricting the back of your throat, creating a soft, soothing sound reminiscent of ocean waves. Practice this tranquil technique 5-10 times to enhance focus and mindfulness.

**Belly Breathing:** Sit comfortably with a straight back. Place one hand on your chest and the other on your belly. Inhale deeply through your nose, allowing your belly to expand while keeping your chest still. Exhale slowly through your mouth, drawing your belly inward. Continue for a few minutes, focusing on the gentle rise and fall of your belly to promote relaxation and ease stress.

**Ocean Sounding Breath:** Sit upright with relaxed shoulders. Inhale slowly through your nose, then exhale through your nose while gently constricting the back of your throat. Aim for a soft, whisper-like sound during both inhalation and exhalation, similar to fogging a mirror. Repeat this calming exercise ten times to cultivate a sense of peace and clarity.

**Humming Breath (Calming, Stress Relief):** Close your eyes and take a slow, deep breath through your nose. Exhale slowly through your mouth while humming softly. Repeat this soothing practice 5-10 times to calm your mind and release tension.

**Day 17 Warm-Ups Routine:**

You will know these movements by now, so we will stop the diagrams for the warm-ups to improve the speed of your workout.

**Shoulder Rolls, Neck Tilts, Ankle Pumps, Wrist Circles, Side Stretch, Chair March, and Seated Rowing.**


**Day 17 Main Sequence: Flow and Strength**

**Chair Warrior Sequence: Embrace Your Inner Warrior**

Warrior 1

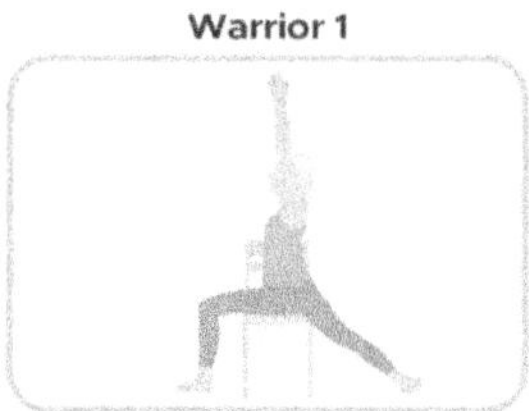

**Warrior 1:** Begin by sitting sideways on the chair with your right leg bent in front of you and your left leg extended back. Inhale deeply as you straighten the left leg as much as possible. Keep your torso over the right leg and lift your arms up towards the ceiling. Feel the power and stretch in your body as you hold this pose.

Warrior 2

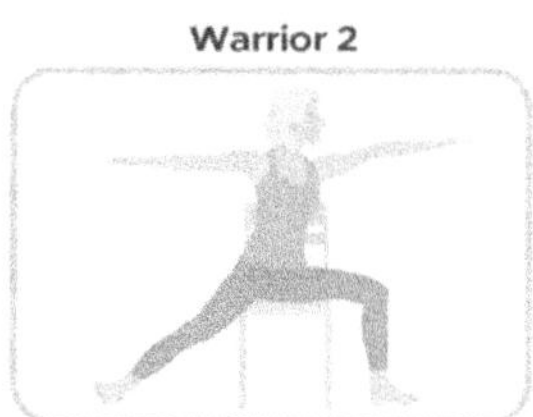

**Warrior 2:** With a smooth transition, turn your torso to face the front of the chair. Extend your arms out to the sides, palms facing down. Take deep breaths, feeling the strength and stability in your legs and core. Inhale and exhale deeply three times, grounding yourself in the moment.

Reverse Warrior

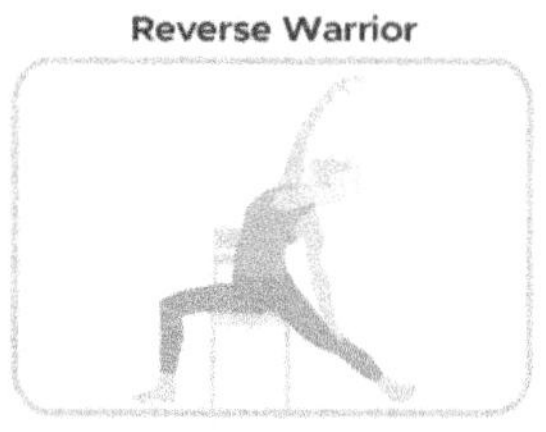

**Reverse Warrior:** Flowing effortlessly from Warrior 2, gently move your left hand down towards your left foot. Lift your right hand up and slightly over your head, opening up the chest and side of the body. Hold this energizing pose for 10-15 seconds, breathing deeply and repeating on the opposite side. If needed, take a brief rest to recharge before continuing.

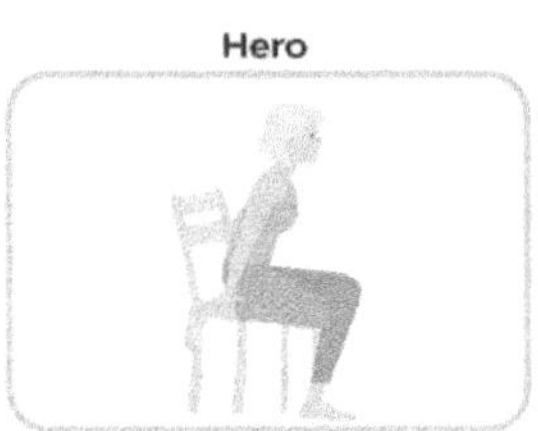



**Hero's Pose: Graceful Strength:** Slide to the front edge of your seat and extend your left leg back, keeping the knee bent. Ensure your bent knee points downwards, with your foot flat against the side of the chair. Breathe deeply, holding this dignified pose for 3-5 breaths. Feel the stretch and empowerment in your body. Return to a neutral position and repeat on the opposite leg, embracing the heroic feeling in your stance.

By integrating these poses into a flowing sequence, you'll cultivate both strength and serenity, transforming your practice into a seamless and empowering experience.

**Day 18 Warm-Ups Routine:**

You will know these movements by now, so we will stop the diagrams for the warm-ups to improve the speed of your workout.

**Shoulder Rolls, Neck Tilts, Ankle Pumps, Wrist Circles, Side Stretch, Chair March, and Seated Rowing.**

**18 Main Sequence: Harmony and Strength**

Seated Eagle

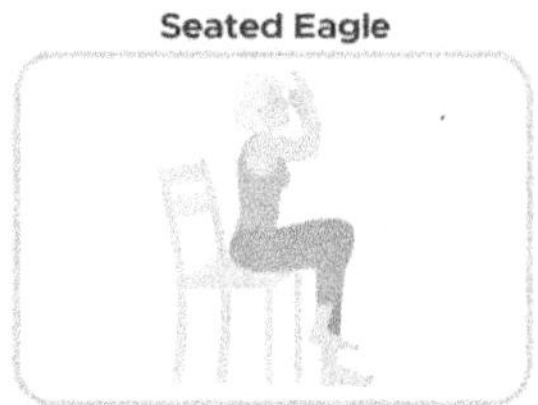

**Seated Eagle Pose: Unite and Balance:** Begin by sitting upright in your chair with your feet firmly planted on the floor. Bring your hands together in front of your chest, elbows bent, and twist your right arm under your left, touching your palms together. Keep your spine tall and shoulders relaxed. Cross your right leg over your left, finding your balance. Inhale deeply through your nose, holding the pose for three breaths. Exhale slowly through your mouth. Repeat this calming pose three times before gently releasing.

Tree-Advanced

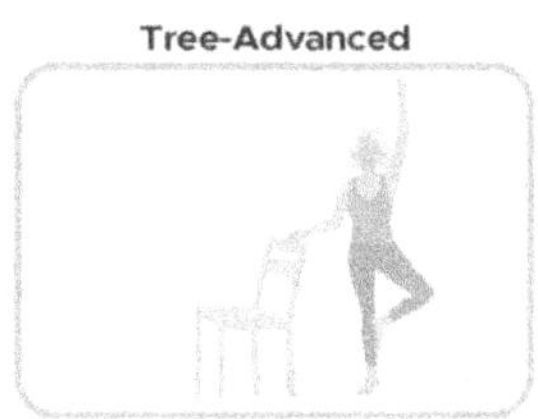

**Tree Pose: Rooted Grace:** Stand beside your chair, holding onto the backrest with your right hand for support. Place your right foot flat on the ground. Lift your left foot and position it against the inner thigh or calf of your right leg, avoiding the knee. Extend your left arm overhead, fingertips reaching towards the sky. Feel your body align and hold the pose for 5-10 deep breaths. Find your center of gravity and focus. Repeat on the opposite side to enhance balance and stability.

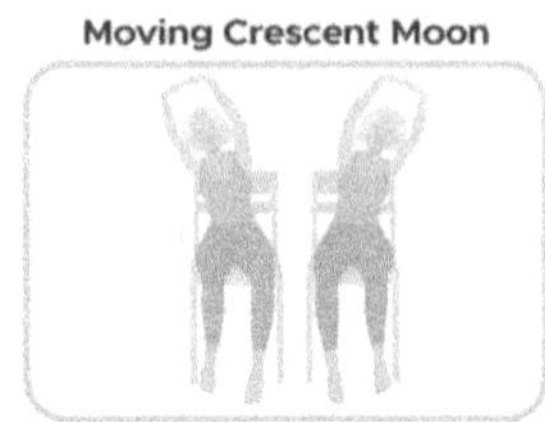



**Moving Crescent Moon Pose: Flowing Elegance:** Sit upright in your chair and stretch both arms overhead, interlocking your fingers. Lean gracefully to the right, enjoying the stretch along your side. Inhale deeply as you return to center, exhale. Repeat this gentle sway to the left, feeling the soothing rhythm of your breath. Continue this fluid motion five times, embracing the tranquil cadence of movement and breath.

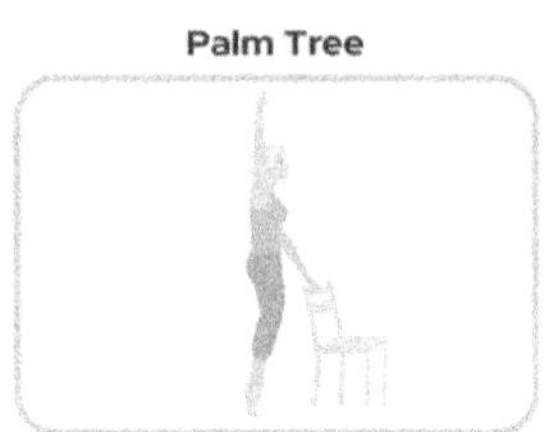



**Palm Tree Pose: Reach for Radiance:**Stand facing the back of the chair, holding onto the backrest with your left hand. Rise onto the balls of your feet and extend your right arm overhead, elongating the side of your body. Feel the stretch and strength in your calf muscles. Return your hand to the chair and ground your feet. Switch sides, holding onto the backrest with your right hand. Rise onto your toes and extend your left arm overhead, luxuriating in the stretch along your side. Hold for 3-5 seconds, then relax. This pose cultivates balance and flexibility with each graceful extension.

By harmonizing these poses, you'll cultivate strength, balance, and a sense of fluidity in your practice, embodying grace and poise with each movement.

**Day 19 Warm-Ups Routine:**

You will know these movements by now, so we will stop the diagrams for the warm-ups to improve the speed of your workout.

**Shoulder Rolls, Neck Tilts, Ankle Pumps, Wrist Circles, Side Stretch, Chair March, and Seated Rowing.**

**19 Main Sequence: Breath, Stretch, and Balance**

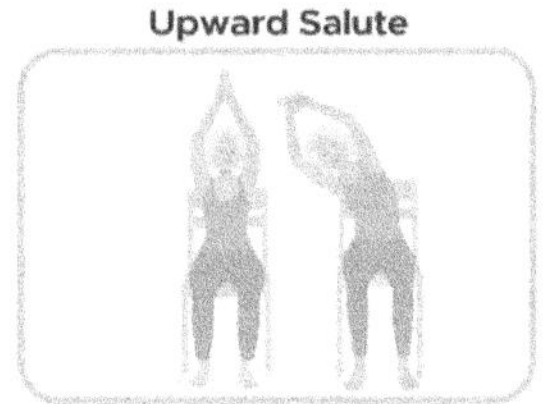


**Upward Salute: Reach for the Sky:** Sit upright with your feet planted firmly on the floor. Inhale deeply, extending your arms overhead with palms facing each other. Feel the stretch through your hips, back, and shoulders as you hold the pose for three to five steady breaths. Gaze straight ahead or lift your eyes towards the heavens. Exhale slowly as you lower your arms, grounding yourself back into the present moment.

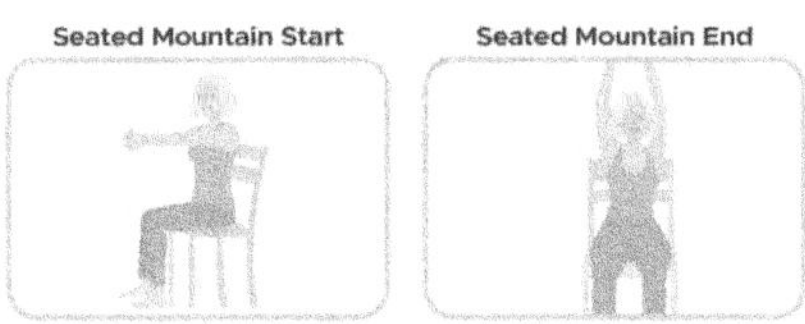

**Seated Mountain Posture: Align and Extend:** Maintain your seated position with feet flat on the floor. Inhale deeply as you extend your arms outwards, interlocking your fingers and turning your palms outward. Lift your hands towards the ceiling, aligning your head, trunk, and hands in a harmonious line. Feel the lengthening in your spine and engage your core. Hold this powerful stance for 3-5 breaths, soaking in the rejuvenating energy that flows through your uplifted posture.

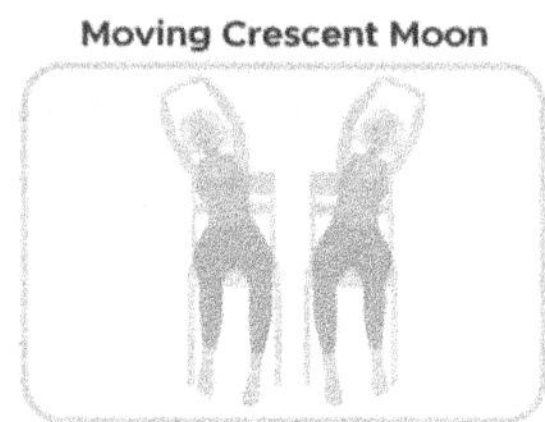


**Crescent Moon Posture: Flowing Grace:** Sit tall in your chair and extend your left arm overhead, creating a graceful "Y" shape. Lean gently to the right, stretching your side body and feeling the expansion in your core. Inhale deeply as you return to center, exhale. Repeat this elegant sway to the left, extending your right arm overhead in a radiant "Y" shape. Hold each side for two breaths, inhale, and exhale as you return to center. Flow through this crescent moon posture five times, embodying fluidity and balance with every movement.

**Purification Breathing: Revitalize and Balance:** Find comfort with your back straight and feet grounded. Place your hands on your knees and close your eyes if preferred. Inhale deeply through your nose, allowing your chest and abdomen to expand with rejuvenating energy. Exhale forcefully yet controlled through your mouth, drawing your abdomen inwards to expel any stagnant energy. Repeat this purifying breath cycle for several rounds, feeling renewed vitality and restored equilibrium wash over your entire being.

This sequence harmonizes breath, movement, and alignment, guiding you towards inner balance, strength, and rejuvenation with each deliberate posture.

**Day 20 Warm-Ups Routine:**

You will know these movements by now, so we will stop the diagrams for the warm-ups to improve the speed of your workout.

**Shoulder Rolls, Neck Tilts, Ankle Pumps, Wrist Circles, Side Stretch, Chair March, and Seated Rowing.**

**20 Main Sequence: Stretch, Flex, and Engage**

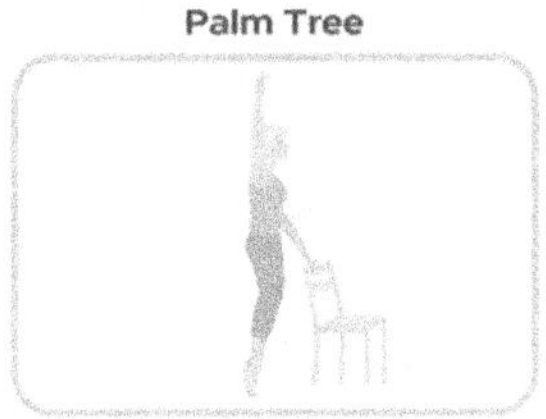


**Palm Tree Pose: Stretch to the Sky:** Stand facing the back of the chair, holding onto the backrest with your left hand. Rise onto the balls of your feet and extend your right arm overhead, feeling the stretch along the side of your body. Return your hand to the chair and flatten your feet. Repeat with the opposite arm: hold onto the backrest with your right hand, rise onto the balls of your feet, and extend your left arm overhead. Hold for 3-5 seconds, then return to normal. This pose tones your calves, legs, knees, back, and neck while improving balance.

Pike Pulse

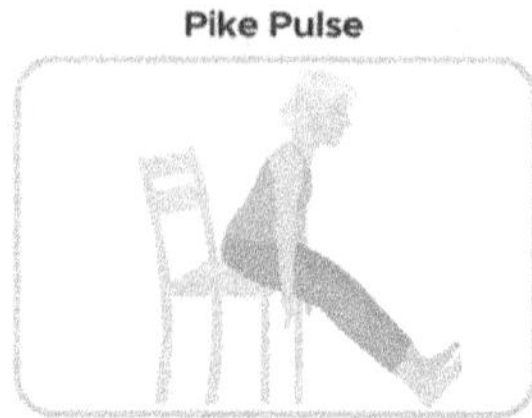

**Pike Pulse: Power Up Your Core:** Sit towards the edge of the chair and extend both legs straight out in front. Place your hands on the armrests or sides of the chair for support, or keep them beside you. Engage your abs and pulse your legs upwards, lifting them slightly off the ground and back down. Perform ten pulses, keeping your core engaged throughout to work your abs, obliques, and lower back.

Seated Eagle

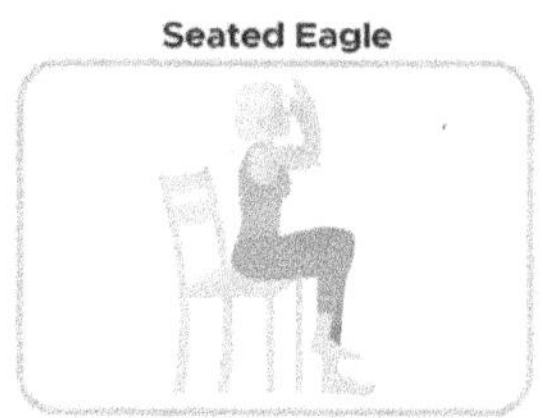

**Seated Eagle Pose: Embrace the Eagle:** Sit straight with your feet flat on the floor. Cross your right thigh over your left thigh. Inhale through your nose, extend your arms in front, and cross your right arm over your left. Exhale slowly. Inhale again and bend your elbows, bringing your palms together. Hold the pose for 5-10 breaths, feeling the stretch in your wrists, elbows, and shoulder joints. Uncross your arms and legs, then switch sides and repeat: cross your left thigh over your right thigh, extend your arms in front, and cross your left arm over your right. Exhale slowly. Inhale, bend your elbows, and bring your palms together. Hold the pose for 5-10 breaths.

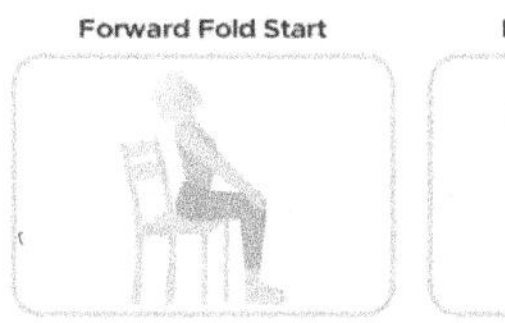
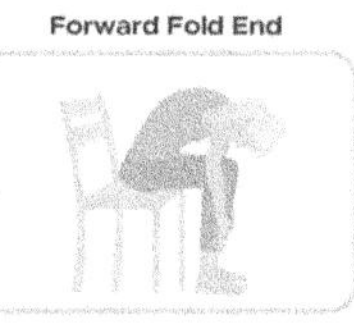

Forward Fold Start

Forward Fold End

**Forward Fold: Dive into Flexibility:** Place your feet flat on the floor and your hands on your knees. Inhale through your nose, lengthening your spine and looking up. Exhale, hinge at the hips, and fold forward, bringing your chest towards your knees. Allow your hands to grasp your lower legs if possible. Hold this pose for 5-10 breaths, increasing your body flexibility as you relax into the stretch.

This sequence guides you through invigorating stretches and engaging movements, ensuring a balanced and revitalizing practice that enhances flexibility, strength, and overall body awareness.

**Day 21 Warm-Ups Routine:**

You will know these movements by now, so we will stop the diagrams for the warm-ups to improve the speed of your workout.

**Shoulder Rolls, Neck Tilts, Ankle Pumps, Wrist Circles, Side Stretch, Chair March, and Seated Rowing.**

**21 Main Sequence: Embrace the Power and Flow**

Feel the power as you embark on this exhilarating sequence!

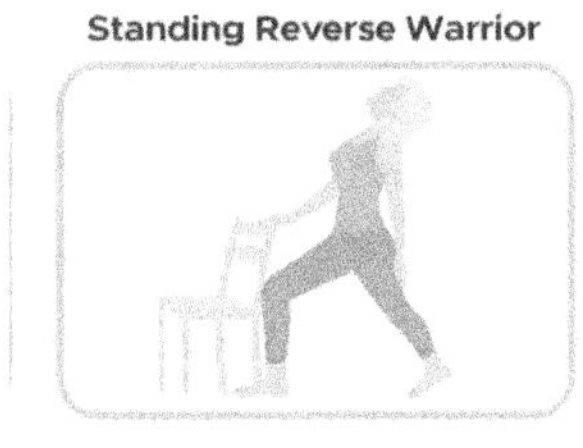

Standing Reverse Warrior

. . .

**Standing Reverse Warrior: Energize Your Spirit:** Stand tall behind the chair, your left hand resting on the backrest, both feet slightly under the chair. Slide your right foot back, bending your left knee until it's nearly parallel to the floor. Extend your right arm out behind you and hold the pose for a thrilling 30 seconds. Switch sides for an electrifying experience. Feel the power surge through you as you embody the warrior within.

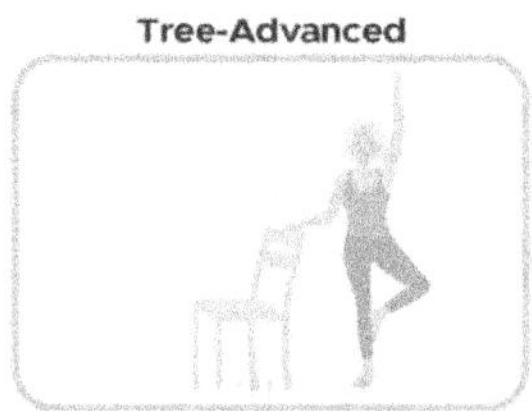


**Tree Pose: Rooted and Reaching:** Stand beside the chair with your right hand on the backrest. Lift your left foot and place the sole against the inner right thigh or calf, avoiding the knee. Raise your left arm up into a majestic crescent moon shape. Take deep breaths, holding for several heart-pounding moments. Switch sides and repeat twice, feeling the rush of stability and strength as you balance like a tree swaying in the wind.

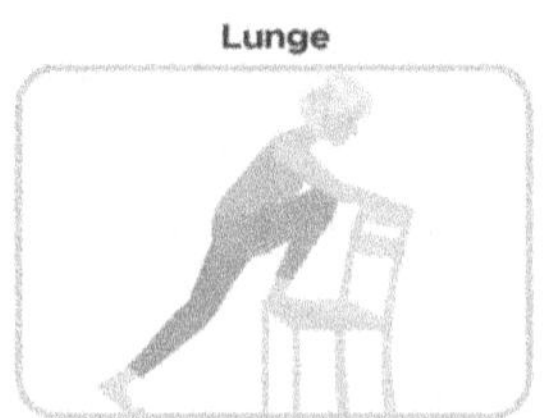

**Lunge: Stretch and Strengthen:** Face the chair seat with both feet flat on the floor, gripping the backrest with both hands. Place your left foot on the chair seat and gently push forward with your right leg, leaning into the stretch of your left leg. Feel the burn as you hold for three breaths, then switch sides for an exhilarating workout. Embrace the dynamic tension as your muscles awaken and strengthen.

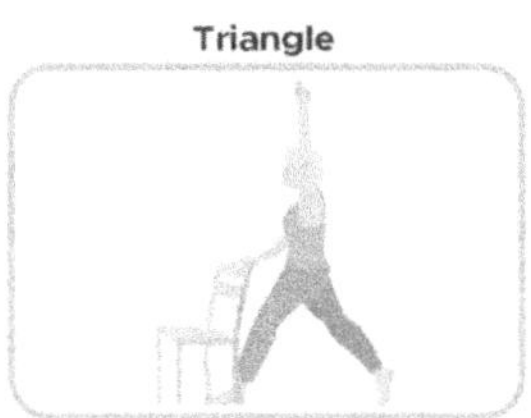


**Triangle: Embrace the Challenge:** Stand beside your chair with the backrest to your right, feet slightly under the chair, and legs shoulder-distance apart. Hold onto the chair back with your right hand, sliding your right foot back about three feet. Extend your left arm up towards the ceiling, breathing deeply and holding for several heart-pounding breaths. Transition to the other side, embracing the challenge and feeling the invigorating stretch as your body forms a powerful triangle.

Embark on this main sequence to ignite your spirit, strengthen your body, and revel in the powerful flow of each pose.

## Day 22-Rest Day/ Mindful Breathing

### Relaxing Breathing Techniques for Focus and Peace

**Box Breathing:** Inhale gently through your nose, counting to four. Hold your breath for four counts. Exhale slowly through your mouth for four counts. Hold the exhale for another count of four. Repeat this rhythmic cycle 5-10 times to promote calmness and center your mind.

**Ocean Breath:** Find a comfortable seated position with relaxed posture. Inhale deeply through your nose, maintaining closed lips. Exhale through your nose while gently constricting the back of your throat, creating a soft, soothing sound reminiscent of ocean waves. Practice this tranquil technique 5-10 times to enhance focus and mindfulness.

**Belly Breathing:** Sit comfortably with a straight back. Place one hand on your chest and the other on your belly. Inhale deeply through your nose, allowing your belly to expand while keeping your chest still. Exhale slowly through your mouth, drawing your belly inward. Continue for a few minutes, focusing on the gentle rise and fall of your belly to promote relaxation and ease stress.

**Ocean Sounding Breath:** Sit upright with relaxed shoulders. Inhale slowly through your nose, then exhale through your nose while gently constricting the back of your throat. Aim for a soft, whisper-like sound during both inhalation and exhalation, similar to fogging a mirror. Repeat this calming exercise ten times to cultivate a sense of peace and clarity.

**Humming Breath (Calming, Stress Relief):** Close your eyes and take a slow, deep breath through your nose. Exhale slowly through your mouth while humming softly. Repeat this soothing practice 5-10 times to calm your mind and release tension.

**Day 23 Warm-Ups Routine:**

You will know these movements by now, so we will stop the diagrams for the warm-ups to improve the speed of your workout.

**Shoulder Rolls, Neck Tilts, Ankle Pumps, Wrist Circles, Side Stretch, Chair March, and Seated Rowing.**

**23 Main Sequence: Experience the Exhilarating Flow**

Feel the rush as you embark on this dynamic sequence!

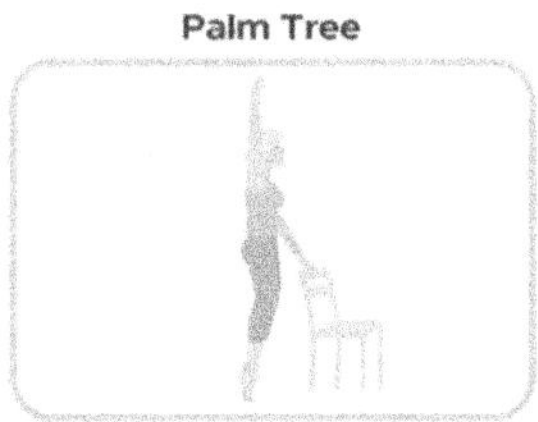

Palm Tree

**Palm Tree Pose - Embrace Balance and Flexibility:** Start by standing facing the back of the chair, gripping the backrest with your left hand. Rise onto the balls of your feet and extend your right arm overhead, stretching the side of your body. Ground your feet and return your hand to the chair. Repeat with the opposite arm: hold onto the backrest with your right hand, rise onto the balls of your feet, and extend your left arm overhead. Hold for an exhilarating 3-5 seconds before returning to normal. This pose challenges your balance while sculpting your calf muscles and stretching your side body.

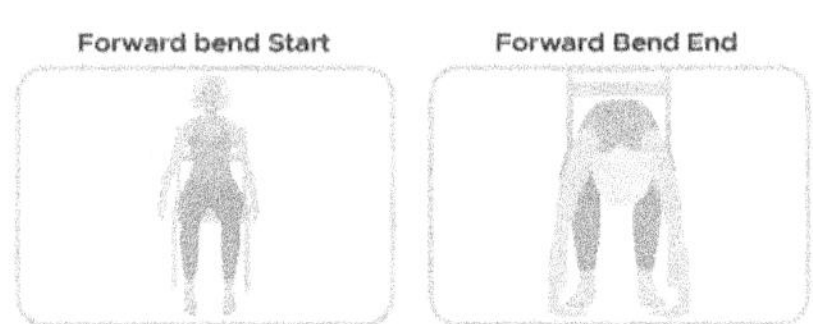

Forward bend Start          Forward Bend End

**Forward Bend - Unlock Your Body's Potential:** Sit up tall and inhale slowly through your nose, extending your arms overhead. Exhale through your mouth as you bend forward from the waist, reaching your hands towards your feet with palms facing up. Feel the stretch and hold for an electrifying ten breaths. To prevent inversion, only bend halfway, keeping your head aligned with your heart. Return to the neutral position, ready to conquer more.

Single Leg Balance

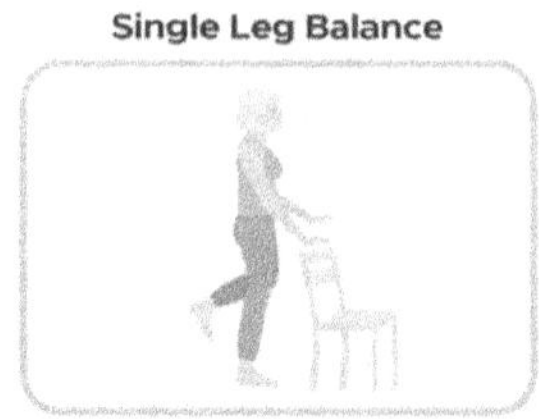

**Single Leg Balance - Find Your Center of Gravity:** Stand behind the chair with your hands lightly resting on the backrest and your feet firmly planted. Lift your left foot off the ground, bending at the knee. Release the chair and focus on maintaining your balance. Hold for an electrifying 5-10 seconds before repeating on the

**Day 24 Warm-Ups Routine:**

**Shoulder Rolls, Neck Tilts, Ankle Pumps, Wrist Circles, Side Stretch, Chair March, and Seated Rowing.**

**24 Main Sequence: Unleash Your Inner Strength**

Feel the power and energy flow through you with each pose in this exhilarating sequence!

Moving Crescent Moon

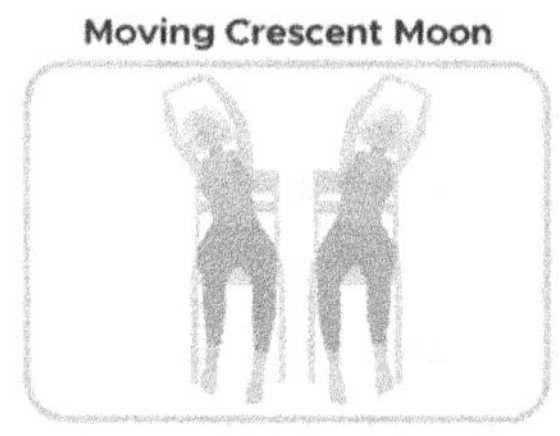

**Crescent Moon - Reach for the Sky:** Sit up tall in your chair and stretch your left arm overhead in a triumphant 'Y' shape. Lean your body to the right and hold for two breaths. Inhale while returning to the center, then exhale. Now, switch to the other side. Stretch your right arm overhead in a victorious 'Y' shape and lean your body to the left. Hold for two breaths before returning to the center. Repeat the left-right stretch for a thrilling experience.

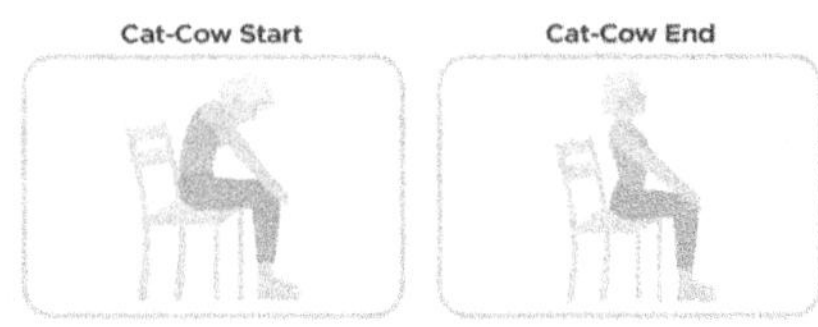



**Cat-Cow Pose - Mobilize Your Spine and Open Your Heart:** Sit up straight in your chair, inhale, and place your hands on your knees. Exhale while rounding your back and tucking your chin towards your chest. Hold the pose for a thrilling five breaths. Inhale, slowly arch your back, and lift your chin and chest upwards. Hold for a victorious moment before exhaling. Alternate between these poses for an electrifying 5-10 breaths.

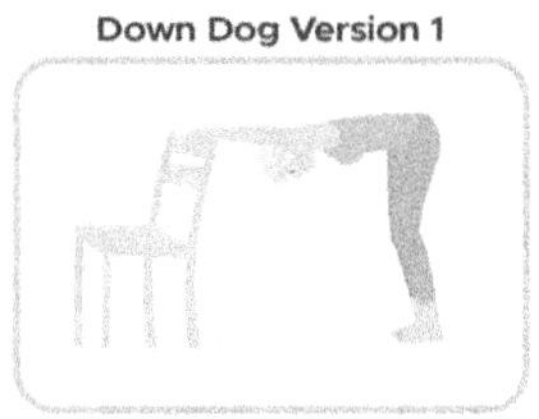



**Down Dog Version 1 - Strengthen Your Core and Spine:** Stand facing the back of your chair, arms-length away. Spread your fingers wide and place them on the back of the chair. Step your feet back until your arms are stretched out straight, forming an inverted 'V' with your body. Push your hips back and up, keeping your feet firmly planted on the floor. Stay in this pose for 3-5 breaths before repeating. Feel the power surging through your core and spine.

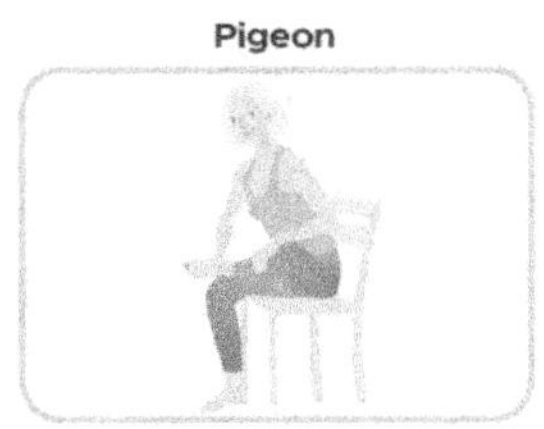

**Pigeon Pose - Enhance Your Mobility and Release Tension:** Sit upright with both feet planted on the floor. Lift your left ankle and place it over your right thigh, creating a majestic figure-four shape. Point your left knee outwards as much as possible. If comfortable, gently press down on the left knee for a deeper stretch. For an even deeper stretch, hinge at the hips and lean forward slightly, keeping your back straight. Hold for several exhilarating breaths before switching sides. Lift your right ankle and place it over your left thigh. Hold for several breaths before releasing. Feel the tension melting away as you surrender to the stretch.

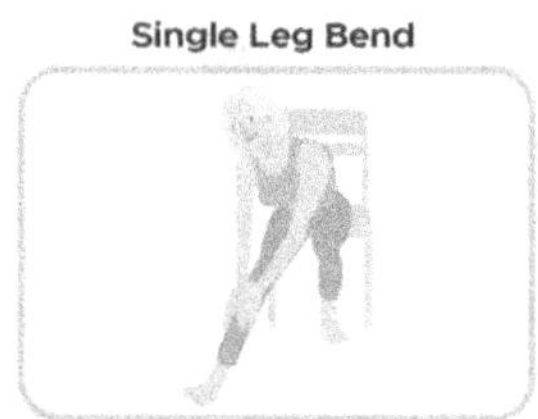

Single Leg Bend

**Leg Forward Bends - Strengthen and Balance:** Sit straight with your feet flat on the ground. Inhale and extend one leg straight in front of you while keeping the other foot planted on the floor. As you exhale, bend forward towards the extended leg, aiming to touch your toes. Hold for three to five breaths before repeating with the opposite leg. Feel the power in your muscles as you stretch and strengthen with each movement.

**Seated Twist - Unlock Your Spine:** Start with your back straight. As you exhale, place your left hand on your right knee and your right hand behind your back or on the chair's backrest. Use your hands to gently twist your upper body to the right. Hold for three breaths, return to the center, and repeat on the other side. As you exhale, place your right hand on your left knee and your left hand behind your back or on the chair's backrest. Gently twist your upper body to the left. Hold for three breaths and return to the center. Feel the exhilaration as you unlock tension and revitalize your spine.

## Day 25 Rest Day/ Mindful Breathing

### Relaxing Breathing Techniques for Focus and Peace

**Box Breathing:** Inhale gently through your nose, counting to four. Hold your breath for four counts. Exhale slowly through your mouth for four counts. Hold the exhale for another count of four. Repeat this rhythmic cycle 5-10 times to promote calmness and center your mind.

**Ocean Breath:** Find a comfortable seated position with relaxed posture. Inhale deeply through your nose, maintaining closed lips. Exhale through your nose while gently constricting the back of your throat, creating a soft, soothing sound reminiscent of ocean waves. Practice this tranquil technique 5-10 times to enhance focus and mindfulness.

**Belly Breathing:** Sit comfortably with a straight back. Place one hand on your chest and the other on your belly. Inhale deeply through your nose, allowing your belly to expand while keeping your chest still. Exhale slowly through your mouth, drawing your belly inward. Continue for a few minutes, focusing on the gentle rise and fall of your belly to promote relaxation and ease stress.

**Ocean Sounding Breath:** Sit upright with relaxed shoulders. Inhale slowly through your nose, then exhale through your nose while gently constricting the back of your throat. Aim for a soft, whisper-like sound during both inhalation and exhalation, similar to fogging a mirror. Repeat this calming exercise ten times to cultivate a sense of peace and clarity.

**Humming Breath (Calming, Stress Relief):** Close your eyes and take a slow, deep breath through your nose. Exhale slowly through your mouth while humming softly. Repeat this soothing practice 5-10 times to calm your mind and release tension.

## Day 26 Warm-Ups Routine:

**Shoulder Rolls, Neck Tilts, Ankle Pumps, Wrist Circles, Side Stretch, Chair March, and Seated Rowing.**

. . .

**Day 26 Main Sequence:**

**Chair Warrior Sequence: Embrace Your Inner Warrior**

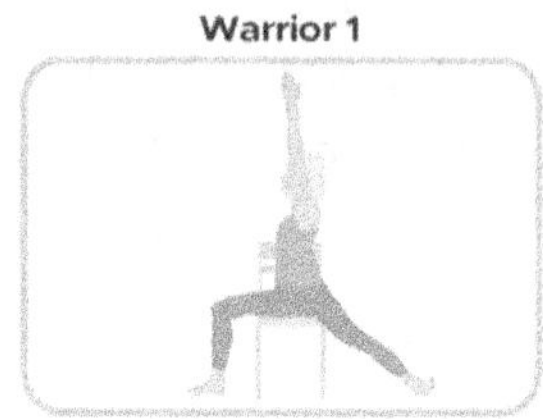


**Warrior 1:** Begin by sitting sideways on the chair with your right leg bent in front of you and your left leg extended back. Inhale deeply as you straighten the left leg as much as possible. Keep your torso over the right leg and lift your arms up towards the ceiling. Feel the power and stretch in your body as you hold this pose.

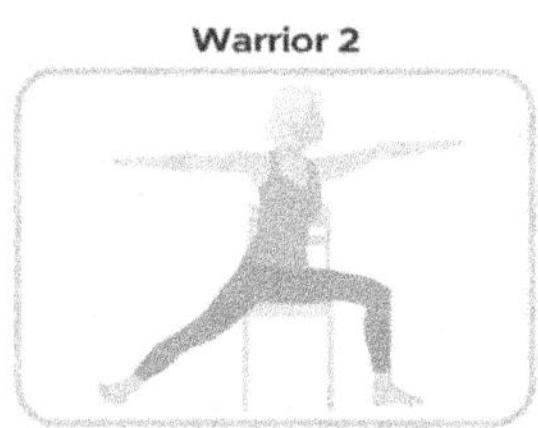


**Warrior 2:** With a smooth transition, turn your torso to face the front of the chair. Extend your arms out to the sides, palms facing down. Take deep breaths, feeling the strength and stability in your legs and core. Inhale and exhale deeply three times, grounding yourself in the moment.

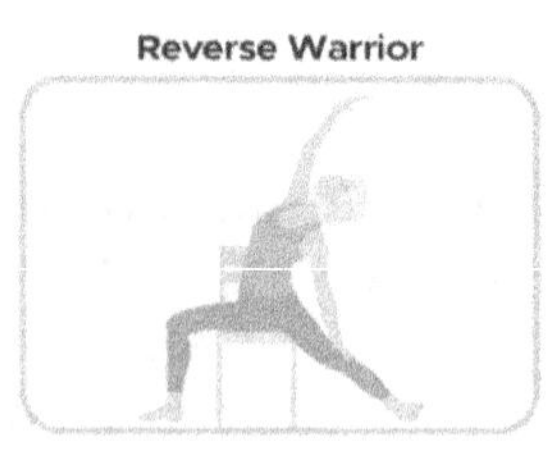

**Reverse Warrior:** Flowing effortlessly from Warrior 2, gently move your left hand down towards your left foot. Lift your right hand up and slightly over your head, opening up the chest and side of the body. Hold this energizing pose for 10-15 seconds, breathing deeply and repeating on the opposite side. If needed, take a brief rest to recharge before continuing.

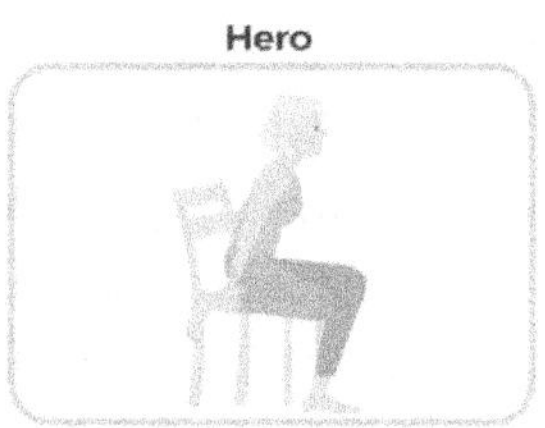



**Hero's Pose: Graceful Strength:** Slide to the front edge of your seat and extend your left leg back, keeping the knee bent. Ensure your bent knee points downwards, with your foot flat against the side of the chair. Breathe deeply, holding this dignified pose for 3-5 breaths. Feel the stretch and empowerment in your body. Return to a neutral position and repeat on the opposite leg, embracing the heroic feeling in your stance.

By integrating these poses into a flowing sequence, you'll cultivate both strength and serenity, transforming your practice into a seamless and empowering experience.

**Day 27 Warm-Ups Routine:**

**Shoulder Rolls, Neck Tilts, Ankle Pumps, Wrist Circles, Side Stretch, Chair March, and Seated Rowing.**

**27 Main Sequence: Embrace the Challenge and Unlock Your Full Potential**

Dive into this energizing sequence and feel the thrill of each pose as you build strength and balance!

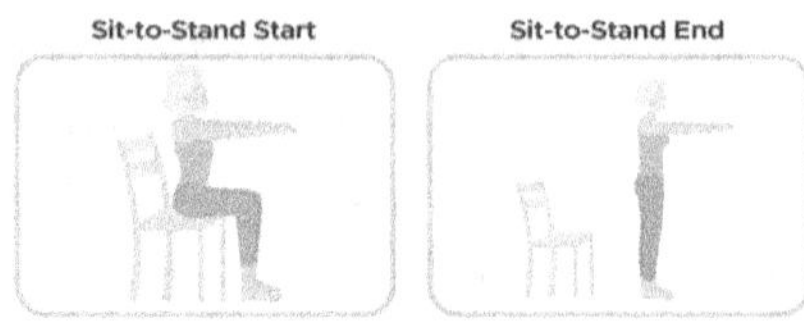


**Sit-to-Stand - Ignite Your Lower Body:** Sit at the front edge of your chair with feet firmly planted on the floor. Place your hands on your thighs or the chair's armrests. Lean forward slightly and push into your hands while straightening your legs to stand up. Slowly reverse the movement to sit back down. Repeat this exhilarating movement 5-10 times in rapid succession. Feel the power surging through your lower body with each stand-up.

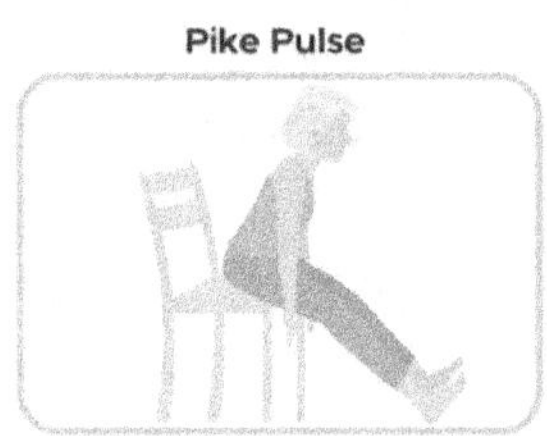


**Pike Pulse - Fire Up Your Abs:** Sit towards the edge of the chair and extend both legs straight out in front. Place your hands on the armrests or sides of the chair for support, or keep them beside you. Engage your abs and pulse your legs upwards, lifting them slightly off the ground and back down. Perform ten pulses, keeping your core engaged throughout. Feel the burn as you activate your abdominal muscles.

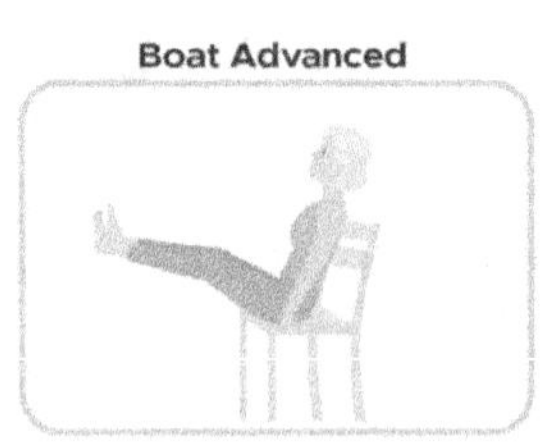

. . .

**Seated Boat Pose - Strengthen Your Core:** Begin by sitting in the middle of your chair with feet flat on the floor. Hold onto the sides of the chair for support. Lean back slightly and lift both feet off the floor, bringing your knees towards your chest. Hold for several exhilarating breaths before lowering your feet back to the ground. Repeat four times, alternating which leg is first on the ground each time. Feel the fire burning in your core as you engage your muscles.

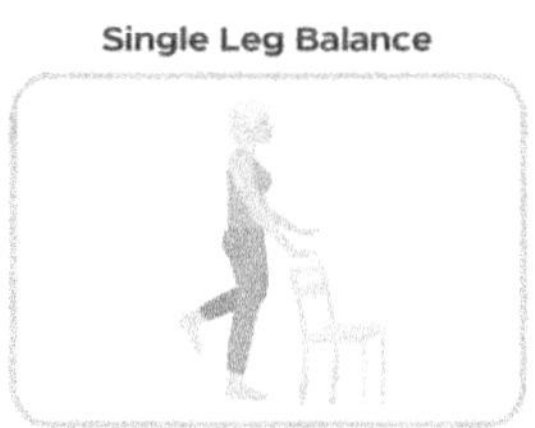


**Single Leg Balance - Find Your Center:** tand behind the chair with your hands loosely on the backrest and feet flat on the floor. Lift your left foot off the ground, bending at the knee. Release the chair and focus on your balance. Hold for an electrifying 10-20 seconds before repeating on the other side. Feel the excitement as you find your center of balance.

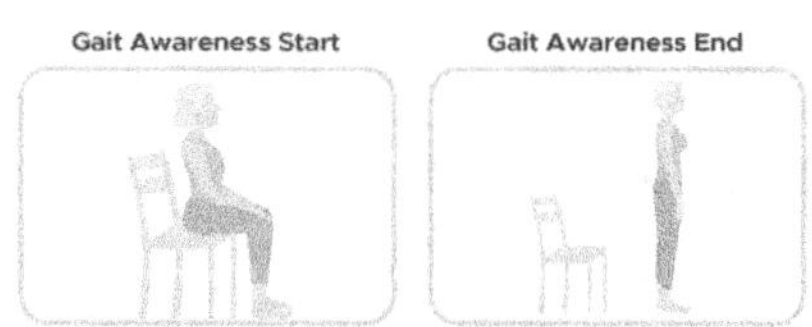


**Gait Awareness Pose - Connect Mind and Body:** seated with your hands on your thighs. Stand up just in front of the chair. Mindfully and slowly lift your right knee towards your chest, then step your right foot forward, placing it down heel first. Shift your weight onto your right foot, lifting your left foot and stepping it forward in the same manner. Continue this slow and deliberate "walking" for several steps, then turn around and repeat in the opposite direction. Feel the connection between your mind and body as you move with intention.

Feel the exhilaration of each movement and embrace the challenge as you unlock your full potential!

## Day 28 Rest Day/ Mindful Breathing

### Relaxing Breathing Techniques for Focus and Peace

**Box Breathing:** Inhale gently through your nose, counting to four. Hold your breath for four counts. Exhale slowly through your mouth for four counts. Hold the exhale for another count of four. Repeat this rhythmic cycle 5-10 times to promote calmness and center your mind.

**Ocean Breath:** Find a comfortable seated position with relaxed posture. Inhale deeply through your nose, maintaining closed lips. Exhale through your nose while gently constricting the back of your throat, creating a soft, soothing sound reminiscent of ocean waves. Practice this tranquil technique 5-10 times to enhance focus and mindfulness.

**Belly Breathing:** Sit comfortably with a straight back. Place one hand on your chest and the other on your belly. Inhale deeply through your nose, allowing your belly to expand while keeping your chest still. Exhale slowly through your mouth, drawing your belly inward. Continue for a few minutes, focusing on the gentle rise and fall of your belly to promote relaxation and ease stress.

**Ocean Sounding Breath:** Sit upright with relaxed shoulders. Inhale slowly through your nose, then exhale through your nose while gently constricting the back of your throat. Aim for a soft, whisper-like sound during both inhalation and exhalation, similar to fogging a mirror. Repeat this calming exercise ten times to cultivate a sense of peace and clarity.

**Humming Breath (Calming, Stress Relief):** Close your eyes and take a slow, deep breath through your nose. Exhale slowly through your mouth while humming softly. Repeat this soothing practice 5-10 times to calm your mind and release tension.

Embrace the excitement and energy of each breath, empowering yourself to conquer every challenge with renewed vitality and determination!

Congratulations! You've made it through day 28! Feel the pride and accomplishment as you reflect on your journey. Take a moment to celebrate your achievements and embrace the transformation within you.

**We have ended the routine on a rest day because tomorrow is the day to retest yourself and see how much improvement you have made. Aim to double your score on all of the tests and get ready to surprise yourself with how much you've improved.**

The journey may be over, but the adventure continues. Keep exploring, keep growing, and keep thriving!

**Important Notes**

So, here we are, at the final chapter of this incredible journey. But let me tell you, this isn't the end – it's just the beginning of your adventure towards greater mobility, strength, flexibility, and balance.

This book is more than just words on paper; it's a catalyst for transformation. It's about embracing the art of graceful aging by taking deliberate steps towards balance and well-being. It's about seizing each day with gusto, optimizing both your physical and mental health.

Now, the torch has been passed to you. You've been equipped with the tools, the roadmap to a better life as you journey through the years. It's like a compass pointing towards a horizon brimming with endless possibilities. Embrace it wholeheartedly, savoring every moment, and watch as a vibrant, fulfilling aging process unfolds before you.

The canvas of your life lies before you, blank and waiting to be painted. And with the techniques and wisdom you've gained, I have no doubt that each stroke will be a masterpiece of balance, vitality, and grace.

our mission is to champion wellness, one stage of life at a time. It would be an honor to hear how these steps have made a meaningful difference in your life. Feel free to share your experiences and leave an honest review on Amazon. Your words will not only be an encouragement but also a guiding light for others on a similar path.

Remember, this isn't the end – it's just the beginning of an extraordinary journey towards a healthier, happier you. Let's paint this canvas of life together, creating a masterpiece of vitality and well-being.

# References and Citations

References are in Alphabetical Order

Aaa1badm, & Aaa1badm. (2021a). Guide to Managing Elderly Chronic Pain |

AAA1B. AAA1B. https://aaa1b.org/elderly-chronic-pain/

Basic Facts about Balance Problems | Aging & Health A-Z | American Geriatrics Society | HealthInAging.org. (n.d.). https://www.healthinaging.org/a-z-topic/balance-problems/basic-facts#

Chair Yoga for Balance and Overall Well-Being – HARTZ Physical Therapy. (n.d.). HARTZ Physical Therapy. https://www.hartzpt.-

com/post/chair-yoga-for-balance-and-overall-well-being/#:~:text=A%20recent%20study,gentle%20and%20breathe

Chalicha, E., & Grebeniuk, I. (2023). Chair Yoga Benefits: 8 reasons why you should do seated Exercises. BetterMe Blog. https://betterme.-world/articles/chair-yoga-benefits/#

Cso. (2021). Management For Chronic Pain In Older Adults: Tips That Help. Center for Spine and Ortho. https://centerforspineandortho.-com/news/management-for-chronic-pain-in-older-adults

https://slscommunities.com/funny-quotes-about-aging-gracefully/

9agnino, A. P. A., & Campos, M. M. (2022). Chronic pain in the elderly: Mechanisms and Perspectives. Frontiers in Human Neuro-science, 16. https://doi.org/10.3377/fnhum.2022.3344FF

9epartment of Health & Human Services. (n.d.). Aging - muscles bones and joints. Better Health Channel. https://www.betterhealth.vic.gov-.au/health/conditionsandtreatments/ageing-muscles-bones-and-joints#

9unkin, M. A. (2007, September 30). Sarcopenia with aging. WebMD. https://www.webmd.com/healthy-aging/sarcopenia-with-aging#

First study to show chair yoga as effective alternative treatment for osteoarthritis. (2011, January 11). ScienceDaily. https://www.sci-encedaily.com/releases/2011/01/110111071131.htm#

· · ·

Sletcher, S. (2023, May 30). Potential causes of stiff joints and what to do about them. https://www.medicalnewstoday.com/articles/321KFF#

Sreiberger, E., Nieber, C., & Rob, R. (2020). Mobility in Older Community-Dwelling Persons: A Narrative review. Frontiers in Physiology, 11. https://doi.org/10.3377/fphys.2020.00101

Haigler, H. (2023). The top benefits of chair yoga – yoga for all humans. Yoga for All Humans. https://yogaforallhumans.com/blog/benefits-of-chair-yoga#

Harvard Health. (2011, April 27). Yoga for pain relief. https://www.health.harvard.edu/alternative-and-integrative-health/yoga-for-pain-relief

Harvard Health. (2014a, February 17). Preserve your muscle mass. https://www.health.harvard.edu/staying-healthy/preserve-your-muscle-mass#:~:text=Age%29related%20muscle,falls%20and%20fractures.

Harvard Health. (2014b, February 17). Preserve your muscle mass. https://www.health.harvard.edu/staying-healthy/preserve-your-muscle-mass#:~:text=The%20power%20of,not%20just%20strength

How the Aging Brain Affects Thinking. (n.d.). National Institute on Aging. https://www.nia.nih.gov/health/how-aging-brain-affects-thinking#

Howland, S. (2022). Mayo Clinic Minute: Helping older adults manage chronic pain. Mayo Clinic News Network. https://newsnetwork.mayoclinic.org/discussion/mayo-clinic-minute-helping-older-adults-manage-chronic-pain/

· · ·

Bertapati, Y., Nahar, S., & Vursasi, A. Y. (2015). The effects of chair yoga with spiritual intervention on the functional status of older adults. Enfermería Clínica, 28, 310-313. https://doi.org/10.1016/s1130-8621(15)30070-6

Lau, C., Yu, R., & Joo, S. (2015). Effects of a 12-Week hatha yoga intervention on cardiorespiratory endurance, muscular strength and endurance, and flexibility in Hong Kong Chinese adults: a controlled clinical trial. Evidence-based Complementary and Alternative Medicine, 2015, 1-12. https://doi.org/10.1155/2015/781281

Befavour, C. (2020). 3 misconceptions and 3 fun facts about chair yoga – Rise & Vibe. Rise + Vibe. https://www.riseandvibeyoga.-com/blog/chair-yoga#

Lifestyle, N. (2021, October 20). Top 10 chair yoga Positions for Seniors [Infographic]. Senior Lifestyle. https://www.seniorlifestyle.-com/resources/blog/infographic-top-10-chair-yoga-positions-for-seniors/#:~:text=Is%20Chair%20Yoga,from%20an%20injury

Lutz, S. (2015, July 10). Chair Yoga: Gentle, Effective Exercise for Osteoarthritis Pain. Health Central. Retrieved September 20, 2023, from https://www.healthcentral.com/condition/osteoarthritis/chair-yoga-gentle-effective-exercise-osteoarthritis-pain#

Madhivanan, P., Drupp, T., Jaechter, R., & Nhidhaye, R. (2021). Yoga for healthy aging: science or hype? Advances in Geriatric Medicine and Research. https://doi.org/10.20700/agmr20210014

· · ·

Madison. (2023, September 12). How To Manage Balance Problems In Seniors + MeetCaregivers. MeetCaregivers. https://meetcaregivers.com/balance-problems-in-seniors/#

Magazine, G. M. -. (2022, October 18). How does breathing affect your brain? Smithsonian Magazine. https://www.smithsonianmag.com/science-nature/how-does-breathing-affect-your-brain-180970780/#

Maintaining mobility and preventing disability are key to living independently as we age. (2020, November 30). National Institute on Aging. https://www.nia.nih.gov/news/maintaining-mobility-and-preventing-disability-are-key-living-independently-we-age#

May, M. (2023a, May 14). 6 Conditions that Lead to Mobility Limitations in Seniors. Home Care Assistance of Amarillo, TX. https://www.homecareassistanceamarillo.com/what-can-cause-my-elderly-parent-to-have-reduced-mobility/#

Neuroscience News. (2022). How breathing shapes our brain. Neuroscience News. https://neurosciencenews.com/breathing-brain-21174/#

Older adults and balance problems. (n.d.). National Institute on Aging. https://www.nia.nih.gov/health/older-adults-and-balance-problems#

PanWeta, E. (2017). Effect of yoga exercise on circulatory system. juniperpublishers.com. https://doi.org/10.170F0/5YP.2017.07.00124

. . .

Physical activity for healthy aging. (2023a, July 4). Centers for Disease Control and Prevention. https://www.cdc.gov/physicalactivity/basics/older-adults

Professional, C. C. M. (n.d.). Sarcopenia. Cleveland Clinic. https://my.clevelandclinic.org/health/diseases/23143-sarcopenia#

Rountree, N., & Rountree, N. (2022). 10 Health Benefits of Yoga For Aging Adults That Will Make You Want to Start Practicing Now. Yoga Journal. https://www.yogajournal.com/yoga-101/10-anti-aging-health-benefits-of-yoga/#

Six Great Plant-Based Foods to Fight Nerve Pain - Neuropathic Therapy Center | Loma Linda University Health. (2022, July 4). https://lluh.org/services/neuropathic-therapy-center/blog/six-great-plant-based-foods-fight-nerve-pain

Statista. (2023, April 10). Prevalence of chronic pain among U.S. adults in 2021, by age. https://www.statista.com/statistics/1170722/chronic-pain-adults-prevalence-by-age-us/

Sobola, M. (2023). *Chair Yoga for seniors over 60: 10-Minute Exercises to Increase Mobility, Maintain Balance, and Improve Flexibility to Give You The Independence You Deserve!*

Ntompər, M., Grodzicki, T., Ntompər, T., Jordliczek, S., Zubiel, M., & Burowska, I. (2017). Prevalence of Chronic Pain, Particularly with Neuropathic Component, and Its Effect on Overall Functioning of Elderly Patients. Medical Science Monitor, 23, 2470-2476. https://doi.org/10.12659/msm.711240

. . .

Telles, N., Nayal, V., Vacht, C. L., Chopra, A., Patel, K., Jnuk, A., Salvi, P., Bhatia, S., Miranpuri, G. N., & Anand, A. (2017). Yoga: Can it be integrated with treatment of neuropathic pain? Annals of Neurosciences, 24(2), 72-81. https://doi.org/10.11588/ans.2017.240203

Ten reasons to do chair yoga | Yoga Alliance. (n.d.). https://www.yogaalliance.org/About-Yoga/Article-Archive/Ten-Reasons-to-Do-Chair-Yoga#

The top reasons for stiff joints in seniors. (n.d.). https://whitneyrehab.com/the-top-reasons-for-stiff-joints-in-seniors/#

Golpî, E., Vazemi, R., & Soltani, N. (2006). Muscle tissue changes with aging. Current Opinion in Clinical Nutrition and Metabolic Care, 9(4), 427-433. https://doi.org/10.1097/01.mco.0000239424.14473.b2

Webtechs. (2021, January 26). *Funny quotes about aging gracefully - SLS Communities*. Senior Living Services. https://slscommunities.com/funny-quotes-about-aging-gracefully/

Why your joints are stiff and how to help them. (n.d.). WebMD. https://www.webmd.com/rheumatoid-arthritis/ss/slideshow-stiff-joints#

Yao, C., Lee, B., Hong, H., & Nu, Y. (2023). Effect of Chair Yoga Therapy on Functional Fitness and Daily Life Activities among Older Female Adults with Knee Osteoarthritis in Taiwan: A Quasi-Experimental Study. Healthcare, 11(1), 102. https://doi.org/10.3390/healthcare11010102